LET FOOD BE YOUR MEDICINE
COOKBOOK

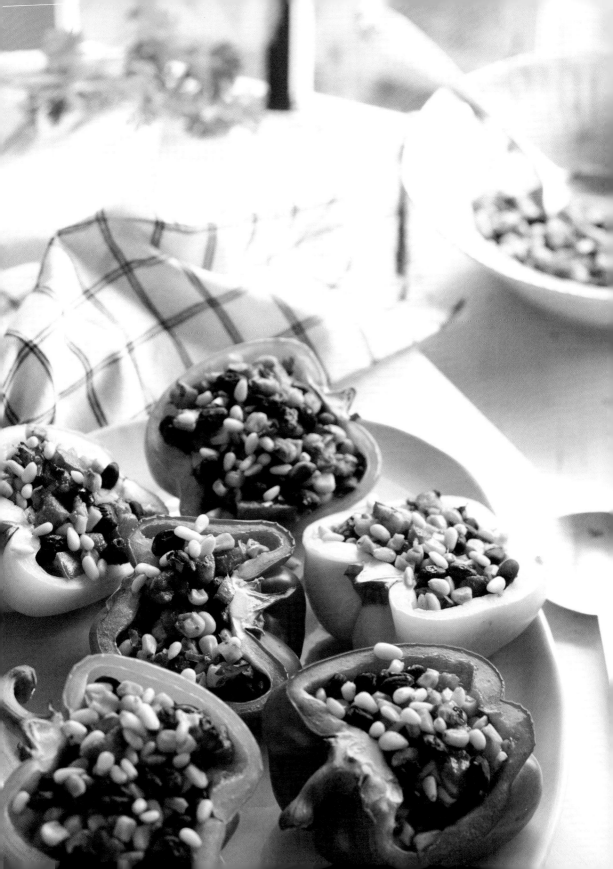

LET FOOD BE
YOUR MEDICINE
COOKBOOK

HOW TO HELP PREVENT
OR REVERSE DISEASE!

DON COLBERT, M.D.

WORTHY®
PUBLISHING

Library of Congress Control Number: 2017954530

For foreign and subsidiary rights, contact rights@worthypublishing.com

Published in association with Ted Squires Agency, Nashville, TN

ISBN: 9781683970576

Recipe Development: Tammy Algood
Food Photography: Mark Boughton Photography
Food Stylist: Teresa Blackburn
Managing Editor: Leeanna Nelson
Additional Photography: istock.com
Interior Design and Typesetting: Bart Dawson
Cover Design: David Carlson, Gilbert & Carlson Design, LLC dba Gearbox

Printed in the United States of America
17 18 19 20 21 LSC 8 7 6 5 4 3 2 1

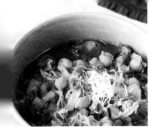

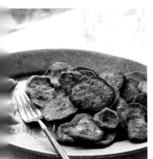

CONTENTS

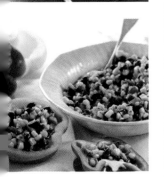

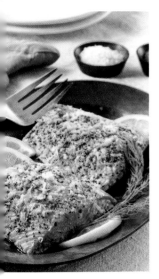

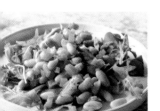

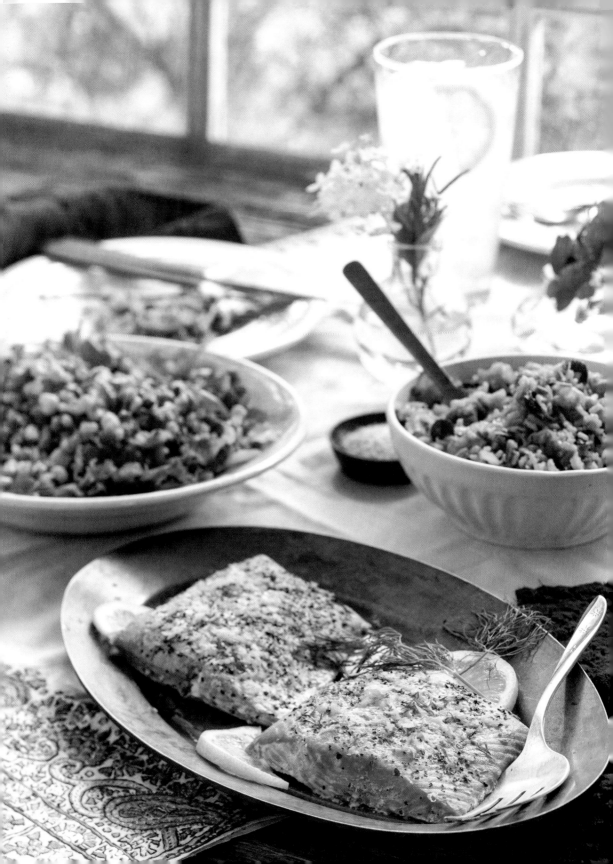

INTRODUCTION

THE MEDITERRANEAN DIET

The Mediterranean Diet mirrors what those living in the Mediterranean actually eat. If you were to investigate, you would find that people in Mediterranean countries do not usually have a membership to a local gym. They usually walk everywhere, including to work. As for eating, it's a big affair with conversation and laughter, and they take their time. Most meals are served with a glass of red wine or bottled water. It is more than just a diet—it is a way of life. In America, we scarf down our food, typically in less than ten minutes and often while driving or watching TV.

Maybe you had a grandmother who said, "Slow down and chew your food!" Those were not wasted words. It is very good advice, and it is something that naturally happens when you enjoy a dinner with others. Chewing your food thirty times is the best for digestion and food absorption. Try it the next time you are eating. If you are chowing down, slow down, put your fork down between bites, and you will probably feel better and have significantly less indigestion and heartburn.

Eating at a slower pace, with friends and family, not only helps you control your appetite, but it also helps reduce your stress. There is nothing wrong with that!

If you want to shift over to the Mediterranean Diet, then there are thirteen important steps to take. Some steps and decisions will be easier than others, but every single step is a good one, except with certain grains. Here is what it usually takes:

1. Eliminate processed foods, which include chips, snacks made with hydrogenated fat, cakes, candies, cookies, crackers, high-sugar cereals, white bread, highly-processed foods, and high-sugar foods.

2. Substitute olive oil for butter, margarine, salad dressings, and other oils. Get rid of other oils, salad dressings, lard, Crisco, other products with hydrogenated fat, as well as polyunsaturated fats including soybean oil, corn oil, sunflower oil, cotton seed oil, and the mono-unsaturated fat, canola oil.
3. Buy only whole-grain items, fresh fruits, fresh vegetables, nuts, and seeds.
4. Cook and bake with whole-grain products.
5. Avoid fried or deep-fried foods.
6. Choose low-fat, plain yogurt, and sweeten with stevia or fresh fruit.
7. Limit cheese to small amounts of Parmesan or Feta mixed with salads or main dishes.
8. Buy fish and poultry more than red meat.
9. Eat red meat very sparingly.
10. Cut out sugary sweets.
11. Enjoy a glass of red wine (caution: may lead to dependence or alcoholism) or sparkling water with lunch or dinner.
12. Walk, bike, and run as much as you can.
13. Slow down and enjoy your dining experience.

The Mediterranean Diet, like the typical "health" pyramid the USDA produces, is built on levels or layers, where you eat the most of the food items at the bottom of the pyramid and the least of the food items at the top. With that in mind, here is how the Mediterranean Diet looks from the bottom up:

Level One: Complex carbohydrates in the form of brown rice, whole-grain rice, whole-grain pasta, and whole-grain bread (the fresher the better). Other possible options include cracked whole wheat (bulgur wheat), couscous, coarse cornmeal (polenta), and potatoes.

Level Two: Fruits, vegetables, nuts, beans, and other legumes. Salads are made of dark green, leafy lettuce, fresh vine-ripened tomatoes, broccoli, spinach, peppers, onions, and cucumbers. The vegetables are often mixed with pasta or rice, used in salads, served as appetizers, or offered as a main or side dish. Fruits are at this level, but are usually a dessert or snack. Nuts are toppings to add flavor and texture. The beans and legumes are usually in soups, added to salads, used as dips (i.e., hummus), or as a main dish.

Level Three: Olive oil, used instead of other oils, butter, margarine, etc. Not only for cooking, it is commonly mixed with balsamic vinegar as a salad dressing.

Level Four: Cheese and yogurt, in small amounts. Freshly grated Parmesan on pasta or a little Feta cheese on a salad is common. Yogurt (about a cup a day) is how milk is usually eaten, and it is low fat or nonfat, usually served with fresh fruit added. Yogurt is also a salad dressing (i.e., mixed with dill, garlic, onion, and cucumbers).

Level Five: Fish, eaten more than other meats, in about 4-ounce portions, several times a week.

Level Six: Chicken, turkey, and eggs. Chicken in 3- to 6-ounce portions a few times a week is common. The meat is usually skinless and added to soups, stews, and other dishes loaded with vegetables. Two to three eggs, with yolks, per week, rotating every three days.

Level Seven: Red meat, in the form of beef, veal, pork, sheep, lamb, and goat, is eaten only a few times a month. It is then often served as a topping to a vegetable, pasta, or rice dish.

> **FACTOID**
>
> GMOs have been linked to thousands of toxic and allergic reactions, thousands of sick, sterile, and dead livestock, and damage to virtually every organ and system studied in lab animals. Choose organic to avoid GMOs, especially with corn and soy.

THE *MODIFIED* MEDITERRANEAN DIET

The Mediterranean Diet is still an incredibly healthy diet, but I've found the need to modify it. Why? Because the raw ingredients of today are not what they used to be. That may sound a little odd, but in its simplest form: most grains and corns have been crossbred, hybridized, or genetically modified.

Dr. William Davis, in his best-selling book, *Wheat Belly*, does an incredible job explaining the changes to wheat and how that affects us today. He says:

Wheat naturally evolved to only a modest degree over the centuries, but it has changed dramatically in the past fifty years under the influence of agricultural scientists. Wheat strains have been hybridized, crossbred, and introgressed to make the wheat plant resistant to environmental conditions, such as drought, or pathogens, such as fungi. But most of all, genetic changes have been induced to increase yield per acre. The average yield on a modern North American farm is more than tenfold greater than farms of a century ago.

And what does it matter? In the health and medical world, it matters for one huge reason: *inflammation.*

What was created to feed the poor, grow faster, need less irrigation, and be hearty is no doubt an engineering marvel! But it is this genetic recoding of wheat that brings about the effects I see in the doctor's office.

In addition to the revised gluten creating inflammation, there are other side effects. Davis also explained how other studies with gluten have found that it can be addictive, and many people have withdrawal symptoms when they go without wheat. It also increases your appetite. This is not good at all, and yet I see it all the time, coming through my office doors in many shapes and sizes.

And when you talk about diabetes, consider the fact that nutritionists more than thirty years ago found that wheat increases blood sugar more than table sugar does! You can see why even the whole wheat bread of the Mediterranean Diet, though it is better than white bread, is still creating havoc among patients who are fighting obesity, diabetes, hypertension, high cholesterol, and a host of other ailments.

The effect of the daily recommended amount of whole grains on my diabetic patients was a good enough reason for me to deviate away from the industry standard. I have had patients check their blood sugars before eating grains, even corn, and then an hour later, see their sugar levels spike 70–120 mg/dl (milligrams per deciliter) higher than their starting levels. That causes a dramatic release of insulin, similar to that of eating sugar. If you are wondering, non-diabetic sugar levels would usually go up only about 20 to 40 points in comparison.

Staying on the "eat six to ten servings a day of bread, cereal, pasta, rice" as the government recommends was not an option. I started modifying the diets of my diabetic patients years ago for this very reason.

The gluten craze is not just for the very small percentage of people who are truly allergic to gluten. I find it very interesting that, according to Dr. David Perlmutter in his best-selling book, *Grain Brain*, "as many as 40 percent of us can't properly process gluten."

The altered (crossbred, hybridized) gluten is wreaking havoc on our health. It really is. And it is exactly that inflammation that causes so much trouble. Why? Because every single degenerative disease has inflammation as the foundation. *Every single one of them.*

When I work with ADHD, ADD, autistic, bipolar, and schizophrenic patients, inflammation also comes directly into play. Dr. Perlmutter points out that "gluten, and a high-carbohydrate diet for that matter, are among the most prominent stimulators of inflammatory pathways that reach the brain."

Wow!

Interestingly, back in 1994, the American Diabetes Association stated that Americans should get 60–70 percent of their calories from carbohydrates. Guess what happened to the number of patients with diabetes? Yes, it went through the roof. But here is where that stat really takes things to the next level: as Dr. Perlmutter notes, "Becoming a diabetic doubles your risk of Alzheimer's disease."

As for corn, the number one crop in the United States, 88 percent of it is GMO (genetically modified organism). These plants have had their DNA altered in a laboratory by genes from other plants, even animals, viruses, or bacteria.

It isn't just corn that is genetically modified. Cottonseed oil (94 percent of what we grow is GMO), soy (93 percent), canola oil (90 percent), papaya (75 percent of Hawaiian papaya), and sugar beets (90 percent, and more than half of sugar sold in the United States comes from sugar beets) are just a few of our staples that are not what they used to be.

It is estimated that between 70 and 85 percent of processed foods that we find in our local grocery stores contain GMO ingredients. The FDA does not require labels to inform you of GMOs in your food, so technically there is no way to be sure of the exact percentage that we consume. Other GMO foods include tomatoes, potatoes, squash, golden rice, animal feed, and even farm-raised salmon.

As you can see, grains and corn, among other raw ingredients, are not even close to what they used to be. One chief side effect of these alterations is the inflammation they cause in our bodies, and I see that on a daily basis.

The best way to avoid GMO foods is to avoid processed foods and/or choose organic foods. Organic foods are not genetically modified.

Coming back to the Mediterranean Diet, I couldn't believe what Dr. Perlmutter wrote. He makes it plain when he states: "If you modify the traditional Mediterranean Diet by removing all gluten-containing foods and limiting sugary fruits and non-gluten carbs, you have yourself the perfect grain-brain-free diet."

Exactly! That is what I have been saying for years. How exactly did we modify the already great Mediterranean Diet to turn it into the best anti-inflammatory diet in the world? In a nutshell, it comes down to avoiding, minimizing, or rotating every four days wheat and corn.

That may seem like a minor alteration, but it's actually a huge shift, one that is bringing healing to thousands of people!

Without further ado, here is the modified Mediterranean Diet:

Level #1: Fruits, vegetables, nuts, beans, and other legumes. Salads consist of dark green, leafy lettuce, fresh vine-ripened tomatoes, broccoli, spinach, peppers, onions, and cucumbers. Serve vegetables in salads, as appetizers, or as a main or side dish. Fruits are usually a dessert or snack. Use nuts as toppings to add flavor and texture. The beans and legumes are usually in soups, added to salads, used as dips (i.e., hummus), or as a main dish.

Level #2: Steel-cut oats and quinoa, millet or millet bread, brown rice, and sweet potatoes. If you are not gluten-sensitive, trying to lose weight, or suffering from high blood pressure, diabetes, high cholesterol, or another inflammatory disease, then potatoes, sprouted bread (e.g., Ezekiel 4:9 bread), or fermented bread (i.e., sourdough bread) are fine on occasion, rotated every four days, and with moderation (the size of a tennis ball for women and one to two tennis balls for men).

Level #3: Olive oil, used instead of other oils, including butter, margarine, etc. Not only for cooking, it is commonly mixed with balsamic vinegar as a salad dressing.

Level #4: Cheese and yogurt, in small amounts. Freshly grated Parmesan on pasta or a little Feta cheese on a salad is common. Yogurt (about a cup) is how milk is usually eaten, and it is low-fat or nonfat, served with fresh fruit added. Yogurt may also be used as a salad dressing (i.e., mixed with dill, garlic, onion, and cucumbers). Many of my patients are sensitive to dairy and thus may need to minimize, avoid, or rotate it every four days.

Level #5: Fish, eaten more than other meats, in about 4- to 6-ounce portions several times a week. Choose low-mercury fish (see page 63 for a list of mercury in fish).

Level #6: Chicken, turkey, and eggs. Chicken in 3- to 6-ounce portions a few times a week is common. The meat is usually skinless and added to soups, stews, and other dishes loaded with vegetables. Only two to six eggs per week. I recommend organic, pastured eggs with the yolks.

HEALTH

The average American gets 6.9 hours of sleep a night. Too little sleep increases the risk for heart disease, obesity, type 2 diabetes, dementia, accelerated aging, fatigue, depression, and a compromised immune system. We need seven to eight hours a night, consistently.

Level #7: Red meat, in the form of beef, veal, pork, sheep, lamb, and goat, is eaten in 3- to 6-ounce portions once or twice a week or just a few times a month. It is then often served as a topping to a vegetable, pasta, or rice dish. I recommend buying grassfed, organic meat.

Visually in a pyramid form, the Modified Mediterranean Diet, looks like this, with what you eat the most (Level 1) at the bottom and what is recommended you eat the least (Level 7) at the top:

#7
#6#6
#5#5#5
#4#4#4#4
#3#3#3#3#3
#2#2#2#2#2#2
#1#1#1#1#1#1#1

The modified Mediterranean Diet is the best anti-inflammatory diet in the world, but of course, if you are allergic or sensitive to a food (e.g., peanuts, dairy, or fish), then don't eat it. Your revised version has then become your own slightly modified Mediterranean Diet.

It is this very diet—with a few minor adjustments, like avoiding food cravings that lean toward a certain ailment—that is so effective in treating specific illnesses. Quite literally, this modified Mediterranean Diet can usually effectively cure, control, or manage every major disease.

LET FOOD BE YOUR MEDICINE

After thirty years of practicing medicine and fervently looking for answers to my patients' core health issues, the best advice I can give anyone is that they should pursue a diet and lifestyle that provides them with good health, sickness prevention, and the ability to treat actual diseases!

FOODS THAT USUALLY LEAD TO WEIGHT LOSS

1. Green tea
2. Leafy green vegetables
3. Wild salmon
4. Dark chocolate
5. Greek yogurt
6. Berries, lemons, limes, Granny Smith apples
7. Steel-cut oats

The only diet I have found that actually does all this is the modified Mediterranean Diet. It is truly the key to the kingdom of health.

For modifying the modified Mediterranean Diet to a specific disease or ailment, refer to my book, *Let Food Be Your Medicine*. There are dedicated chapters for a special diet and lifestyle for those suffering from cardiovascular diseases, type 2 diabetes, cancer, dementia, ADHD, and mental illness.

You will read about the very tools that will help you treat, cure, control, or manage what ails you. And we are not talking about treating just the symptoms; we are talking about treating the real issues, and I love that as a medical doctor.

The Hippocratic Oath, which all medical doctors swear to uphold, states, "I will prevent disease whenever I can, for prevention is preferable to cure."

Of course prevention is better, which is why the modified Mediterranean Diet is the answer to a long-term lifestyle of health and wellness.

Remember, it was also Hippocrates who said, "Let food be thy medicine and medicine be thy food." We are doing just that! This book is *the* answer to a healthy lifestyle that is also all about prevention. Truly amazing!

I'm so confident this healthy lifestyle is effective at treating any chronic disease that I welcome you to contact my office with what ails you. Together we can come up with a plan of attack that works for you.

Finally, my parting comment is one of hope. I know just how important hope is from when I was a patient myself. Without it, we cannot face tomorrow . . . but with it, we can take on the world.

I want to leave you with hope—a hope that helps you face another tomorrow, hope to grab hold of what you want and not let go, and hope to regain or improve your health.

You can do it!

THE COOKBOOK

This cookbook is unique in that it is organized around a 21-day meal plan. For three weeks, you can make every meal, snack, and dessert in this cookbook, and then you can repeat for weeks on end. The beauty of this meal plan-styled cookbook is you can follow it every 21 days indefinitely, or rotate your favorite recipes into your own set of meals and schedules. It is incredibly versatile! The recipe portion includes full recipes for what is suggested in the meal plan, along with extra recipes that follow the modified Mediterranean Diet. The extra recipes will help you continue this diet plan by giving you different dishes to interchange within the meal plan. Throughout the cookbook, there will be tips, tricks, and suggestions for how to store specific foods, organize your pantry, utilize your freezer, as well as factoids about living a healthy lifestyle.

The shopping lists for each week, found at the beginning of each week's recipes and in Appendix A, will help you get started. They include a list of pantry, freezer, and refrigerator staples, as well as weekly necessary food items to follow the plan. These are made to insure you have the freshest food available for the week.

Your refrigerator is going to be full of lots of fresh produce. It is important to cycle these through your meal plan as much as possible in order to avoid waste. For instance, you will be consuming twice-daily salads that call for plenty of colorful vegetables, so make sure you incorporate the oldest produce in your crisper bin first. If your refrigerator has two crisper drawers, separate the fruits from the vegetables to extend the shelf life of each for as long as possible. Check the produce daily for items that may be starting to deteriorate in quality. You can substitute different fruits or vegetables if you don't like the ones called for in the meal plan. For instance, if a smoothie calls for raspberries, but you don't like them, use an equal portion of another berry that you enjoy and have on hand.

I prefer buying organic produce, however, not everyone can afford organic, and that's okay! Try to choose fresh or frozen fruit and vegetables over canned. For meats and dairy, I prefer grass-fed, or even better is grass-fed, organic meat. For fish, I prefer wild fish instead of farm raised. When cooking in the oven or on the grill using a medium to high heat, choose avocado oil or coconut oil, which both have high smoke points. If cooking at low heat or medium heat, olive oil may be used if for a short period of time. It is best to choose organic, extra-virgin oils, including olive oil, avocado oil, and coconut oil. If salt is included in the recipe, choose Himalayan salt (it is pink in color and can be found at health foods stores) or sea salt. Use grass-fed butter, such as Kerry Gold, which is found at most grocery stores, in place of regular butter. I use organic stevia, such as Pyure stevia, which can be found at most grocery stores. There are a couple of other instances where specific product names are mentioned. These are merely suggestions based on experience, but you may substitute with another brand if desired or preferred.

If you don't have a steamer basket for vegetables, it would be wise to invest in one. Steamed vegetables retain more vitamins and nutrients than those that are boiled or poached. Use the basket with a heavy saucepan that includes a sturdy lid.

These suggested recipes and proposed meals follow the modified Mediterranean Diet and are intended to give you a practical starting point for your own menus, schedules, and health plans. It uses a rotation system of proteins, vegetables, fruits, grains, and nuts to prevent boredom and help your body adjust to your new method of eating. Follow the portion sizes stated carefully for the best success. Use salads and vegetables to keep you full. The meal plan is organized for one individual. The recipes typically make more than one serving, which allows you to properly store extra serving portions to eat at a later time as outlined in the meal plan schedule.

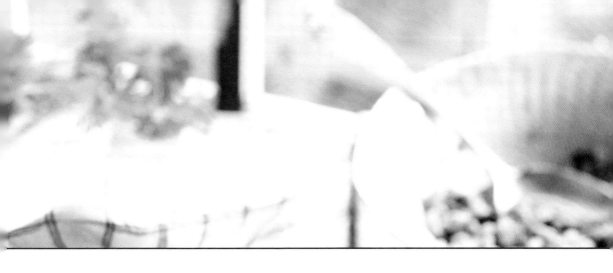

21-DAY
MEAL PLAN

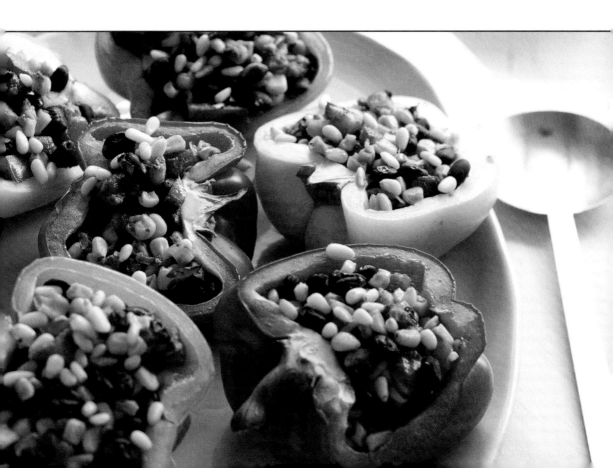

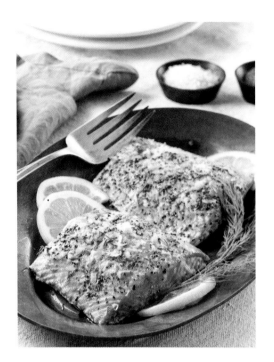

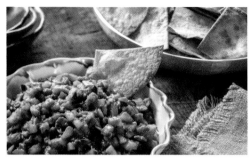

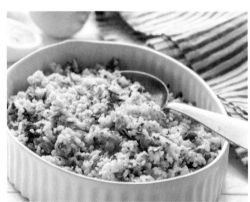

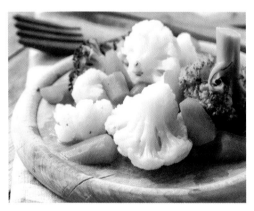

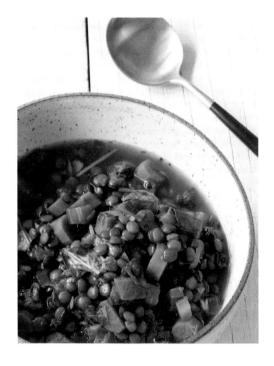

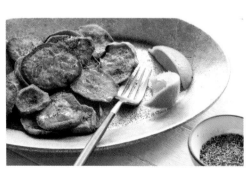

WEEK 1: DAY #1

BREAKFAST (6:00 A.M.):
- 2 slices gluten-free bread, toasted with 1 pat of organic butter, sprinkled with 1 tsp. chia seeds
- 3 oz. turkey sausage (squeeze between two napkins to remove fat)
- ½ cup sliced strawberries
- 1 cup of green tea or coffee, sweetened with stevia, coconut milk for creamer

MID-MORNING SNACK (9:00 A.M.):
- 1 banana

LUNCH (12:00 P.M.):
- Grilled mackerel with tarragon (3-6 oz. for women, 3-8 oz. for men)
- 1 cup broth-based split pea soup
- Oven-roasted eggplant (as much as desired) with chopped fresh oregano
- Large salad with chicory, tomatoes, shredded carrot, and extra-virgin olive oil and balsamic vinegar as dressing (no croutons)
- 1 cup of green tea, water, sparkling water, or unsweetened iced tea with lemon or lime

MID-AFTERNOON SNACK (3:00 P.M.):
- Handful of pecans (approximately 5-10)

....

....

....

....

....

....

....

....

....

....

....

....

....

....

....

....

....

....

....

....

....

....

....

DINNER (6:00 P.M.):

- Grilled turkey tenderloin with fresh chopped thyme and lemon pepper
  (3-4 oz. for women, 3-6 oz. for men)
- Roasted zucchini or butternut squash, mashed and topped with 1 tbsp. chopped pecans
- Steamed green beans with pearl onions (as much as desired)
- Large salad with as many veggies as desired, and extra-virgin olive oil and balsamic vinegar as dressing (no croutons)
- 1 cup of green tea, water, sparkling water, or unsweetened iced tea with lemon or lime

EVENING SNACK (9:00 P.M.):

- Broth-based vegetable soup without potatoes or pasta (½ cup for women, 1 cup for men)

FOOD FACT: BERRIES
(Blackberries, Blueberries, Raspberries, Strawberries)

Storage: Refrigerate always, and if possible, place the berries in a single layer to prevent bruising.

Freeze: Wash and thoroughly drain on paper towels. Cap and core strawberries. Place on a rimmed baking sheet and place in the freezer. When solid, move to a freezer container, label, date, and freeze. There is no need to thaw before using and they keep up to a year.

DAY #2

BREAKFAST (6:00 A.M.):

- Large bowl of steel-cut oatmeal cooked with ground cinnamon and ¼ cup blueberries
- Handful of walnuts (approximately 5-10)
- Smoothie made with 6 oz. coconut, almond, or skim milk, ½ frozen banana, ¼ cup frozen raspberries, strawberries, or blackberries, 1-2 tbsp. ground flaxseeds, 1 scoop plant protein powder, 1 tbsp. cashew nut butter (may add ice or sweeten with stevia to taste)
- 1 cup of green tea or coffee, sweetened with stevia, coconut milk for creamer

MID-MORNING SNACK (9:00 A.M.):

- 1 Granny Smith apple

LUNCH (12:00 P.M.):

- Grilled boneless, skinless chicken breast (3-4 oz. for women, 3-6 oz. for men)
- Black bean soup (½ cup for women, 1 cup for men)
- Steamed spinach (as much as desired) seasoned with a small amount of salt, if desired
- Large salad with Belgian endive, bean sprouts, peppers, and extra-virgin olive oil and balsamic vinegar as dressing (no croutons)
- 1 cup of green tea, water, sparkling water, or unsweetened iced tea with lemon or lime

MID-AFTERNOON SNACK (3:00 P.M.):

- Handful of walnuts (approximately 5-10)

DINNER (6:00 P.M.):

- Extra lean beef (96/4, petite fillet) seasoned with salt or pepper, if desired (3-4 oz. for women, 3-6 oz. for men)
- Steamed broccoli (as much as desired) seasoned with a small amount of salt
- Large salad with sweet corn, lentils, red bell pepper, and extra-virgin olive oil, lime, and balsamic vinegar as dressing (no croutons)
- 1 cup of green tea, water, sparkling water, or unsweetened iced tea with lemon or lime

EVENING SNACK (9:00 P.M.):

- 1 lettuce wrap with 2 oz. chicken, onion, garlic, and other vegetables, seasoned to taste (may add a few slices of avocado)

FOOD FACT: FISH

Flounder has a fine texture and wonderfully delicate flavor. It is enhanced by delicate herbs, such as parsley, chives, thyme, as well as lemon or lime juice and coriander, garlic, and pepper.

DAY #3

BREAKFAST (6:00 A.M.):
- 2-3 eggs (1 yolk, 3 whites) scrambled, poached, or fried (may add onion, mushrooms, and avocado, cooked in olive oil, or a small amount of organic butter)
- Hash browns or sweet potato hash browns (½ cup for women, 1 cup for men) with diced onions and cooked under low heat with olive oil
- ¼ cup raspberries
- 1 cup of green tea or coffee, sweetened with stevia, coconut milk for creamer

MID-MORNING SNACK (9:00 A.M.):
- 1 pear, cored and peeled

LUNCH (12:00 P.M.):
- Grilled flounder with coriander and parsley (3-4 oz. for women, 3-6 oz. for men)
- Roasted sweet potato "fries" with fresh lime juice drizzle (as much as desired)
- ½ cup red beans
- Cucumber and radish salad, topped with Feta and chopped pecans
- 1 cup of green tea, water, sparkling water, or unsweetened iced tea with lemon or lime

MID-AFTERNOON SNACK (3:00 P.M.):

- Raw vegetables of choice with ¼ cup of hummus

DINNER (6:00 P.M.):

- Sliced roasted turkey
  (3-4 oz. for women, 3-6 oz. for men)
- Steamed asparagus with lemon pepper (as much as desired)
- Steamed English peas with pearl onions (as much as desired)
- Large salad with plenty of colorful vegetables and extra-virgin olive oil and balsamic vinegar as dressing (no croutons)
- 1 cup of green tea, water, sparkling water, or unsweetened iced tea with lemon or lime

EVENING SNACK (9:00 P.M.):

- Baked whole apple (unpeeled) sprinkled with ground cinnamon

FOOD FACT: BERRIES
(Blackberries, Blueberries, Raspberries, Strawberries)

Selection: Only purchase berries that are fully ripe. You can tell their ripeness by the color. If the fruit still has slivers of color that don't match the true hue, it's not ripe. And since berries don't continue to ripen after harvest, it's best to avoid purchasing those.

DAY #4

BREAKFAST (6:00 A.M.):
- 1 cup gluten-free cinnamon granola
- Smoothie made with 6 oz. coconut, almond, or skim milk, ½ cup frozen raspberries, 1 banana, 1-2 tbsp. ground flaxseeds, 1 scoop plant protein powder (may add ice or sweeten with stevia to taste)
- 1 cup of green tea or coffee, sweetened with stevia, coconut milk for creamer

MID-MORNING SNACK (9:00 A.M.):
- ½ cup seedless grapes or pitted cherries

LUNCH (12:00 P.M.):
- Grilled salmon with chopped fresh dill (3-6 oz. for women, 3-8 oz. for men)
- 1 cup gluten-free rice noodles with shredded carrot, garlic, chopped fresh parsley, cayenne, extra-virgin olive oil, and black pepper
- Barley vegetable soup (½ cup for women, 1 cup for men)
- Large salad with red leaf lettuce, button mushrooms, seedless grapes, and extra-virgin olive oil and balsamic vinegar as dressing (no croutons)
- 1 cup of green tea, water, sparkling water, or unsweetened iced tea with lemon or lime

MID-AFTERNOON SNACK (3:00 P.M.):

- Handful of unsalted peanuts (approximately 5-10)

DINNER (6:00 P.M.):

- Broiled crab (domestic) cake made with 1 tbsp. light mayonnaise, lemon pepper, cayenne, chopped fresh chives, and a small amount of salt (3-6 oz. for women, 3-8 oz. for men)
- Sweet potato medallions with 1 pat of organic butter (size of 1 tennis ball for women, size of 1-2 tennis ball(s) for men)
- Steamed asparagus (as much as desired)
- Avocado fruit salad, topped with toasted pine nuts, and extra-virgin olive oil, honey, and white wine vinegar as dressing (no croutons)
- 1 cup of green tea, water, sparkling water, or unsweetened iced tea with lemon or lime

EVENING SNACK (9:00 P.M.):

- Celery sticks and ¼ cup gluten-free peanut butter

FOOD FACTS: CANTALOUPES & HONEYDEW

Serving: Both honeydew and cantaloupe are best if served chilled, but not cold. If you prepare it ahead of time, bring it to room temperature at least 15 minutes before serving.

Freeze: Peel and seed the melons, then slice or cube as desired. Place in a freezer container, label, date, and freeze.

DAY #5

BREAKFAST (6:00 A.M.):
- 1 gluten-free bagel, toasted, spread with 1 pat of organic butter, and topped with 1 tsp. toasted, unsalted sunflower seeds
- 1 banana
- 1 cup plain gluten-free Greek yogurt
- 1 cup of green tea or coffee, sweetened with stevia, coconut milk for creamer

MID-MORNING SNACK (9:00 A.M.):
- ½ cup diced cantaloupe or honeydew sprinkled with chopped fresh mint

LUNCH (12:00 P.M.):
- Turkey and flaxseed meatballs, served on thick slices of tomato
- Steamed cauliflower "rice" (as much as desired) with black pepper and a small amount of salt
- Large salad with corn, green onions, pimentos, and extra-virgin olive oil and balsamic vinegar as dressing (no croutons)
- 1 cup of green tea, water, sparkling water, or unsweetened iced tea with lemon or lime

MID-AFTERNOON SNACK (3:00 P.M.):
- 1 tbsp. of unsalted, roasted sunflower seeds

DINNER (6:00 P.M.):

- Boiled large shrimp (8 for women, 12 for men)
- Steamed spaghetti squash noodles with chopped tomato, wilted kale, chives, and 1 tbsp. Feta cheese (as much as desired)
- Large salad with plenty of colorful vegetables and extra-virgin olive oil and balsamic vinegar as dressing (no croutons)
- 1 cup of green tea, water, sparkling water, or unsweetened iced tea with lemon or lime

EVENING SNACK (9:00 P.M.):

- 1 cup steamed edamame pods

FOOD FACTS: SQUASH (SUMMER)

Substitutions: For nearly every recipe except zucchini bread, summer squash varieties can be substituted for each other. This means you can really save money by selecting the type that is most plentiful at the moment.

Selection: Summer squash should be firm and heavy feeling. You don't want to purchase those with obvious skin cracks, soft spots, or ones that have started to look wrinkled.

DAY #6

BREAKFAST (6:00 A.M.):
- 1-2 slices gluten-free bread, toasted and topped with sliced avocado
- ½ broiled grapefruit sprinkled with ½ tsp. chia seeds
- Handful of whole almonds (approximately 5-10)
- 1 cup of green tea or coffee, sweetened with stevia, coconut milk for creamer

MID-MORNING SNACK (9:00 A.M.):
- 1 kiwi, peeled and sliced

LUNCH (12:00 P.M.):
- Veggie burger patty (no bun) topped with tarragon and cayenne (3-4 oz. for women, 3-6 oz. for men)
- Steamed asparagus (as much as desired)
- Large salad with chopped tomato, onion, and carrot pieces, and extra-virgin olive oil and balsamic vinegar as dressing (no croutons)
- 1 cup of green tea, water, sparkling water, or unsweetened iced tea with lemon or lime

MID-AFTERNOON SNACK (3:00 P.M.):
- Handful of whole almonds (approximately 5-10)

DINNER (6:00 P.M.):

- Grilled boneless, skinless chicken breast (3-4 oz. for women, 3-6 oz. for men) with a rub of minced garlic, black pepper, and 1 tbsp. balsamic vinegar
- Roasted summer or winter squash (as much as desired) with fresh thyme, lemon zest, and 1 tbsp. extra-virgin olive oil
- Steamed green beans (as much as desired)
- Large salad with plenty of colorful vegetables and extra-virgin olive oil and balsamic vinegar as dressing (no croutons)
- 1 cup of green tea, water, sparkling water, or unsweetened iced tea with lemon or lime

EVENING SNACK (9:00 P.M.):

- Carrot sticks with ¼ cup spiced lentil dip

FOOD FACTS: SQUASH (WINTER)

Substitutions: When using pureed pumpkin in quick breads, you can substitute equal amounts of pureed butternut squash.

Selection: Because these squash varieties are allowed to fully mature before harvest, it should have a hard and completely firm exterior skin. They should feel heavy for the size.

DAY #7

BREAKFAST (6:00 A.M.):
- ¾ cup gluten-free, high-fiber cinnamon cereal with 8 oz. coconut, almond, or skim milk
- 1 cup diced honeydew or cantaloupe sprinkled with chopped fresh mint
- Handful of cashews (approximately 5-10)
- 1 cup of green tea or coffee, sweetened with stevia, coconut milk for creamer

MID-MORNING SNACK (9:00 A.M.):
- 1 apricot or 8 pitted cherries

LUNCH (12:00 P.M.):
- Grilled turkey breast (3-4 oz. for women, 3-6 oz. for men)
- Chopped cabbage (as much as desired) with shredded carrot and 1 tbsp. light mayonnaise
- Salad greens topped with chopped watermelon, heirloom tomatoes, shallots, cucumbers, and fresh oregano, with extra-virgin olive oil as dressing (no croutons)
- 1 cup of green tea, water, sparkling water, or unsweetened iced tea with lemon or lime

MID-AFTERNOON SNACK (3:00 P.M.):
- Handful of cashews (approximately 5-10)

DINNER (6:00 P.M.):

- Plank grilled whitefish with fresh herb rub (3-6 oz. for women, 3-8 oz. for men)
- Roasted zucchini or butternut squash (as much as desired) with fresh thyme and black pepper
- Steamed cauliflower (as much as desired) with 1 pat of organic butter
- Large salad with plenty of colorful vegetables and extra-virgin olive oil and balsamic vinegar as dressing (no croutons)
- 1 cup of green tea, water, sparkling water, or unsweetened iced tea with lemon or lime

EVENING SNACK (9:00 P.M.):

- 1 veggie lettuce wrap with tomatoes, cucumbers, squash, and cauliflower

FOOD FACT: BANANAS

Freezing: Bananas can be frozen peeled or unpeeled and whole, mashed, or sliced. I like them frozen in slices best because that makes them so much easier to use in smoothies. The important thing to remember is to use ripe bananas rather than those that still have some green showing on the peel. Simply peel, slice, and place in a single layer on a baking sheet lined with parchment paper. Place the baking sheet in the freezer. When the slices are solid, remove and transfer to a freezer container, label, and freeze. There is no need to thaw before using. Just pull the amount you need straight from the freezer.

FOLLOWING AN ANTI-INFLAMMATORY DIET

Over time, from studies, testing, trial and error, experience, and tracking my own patients, I learned that a person following an anti-inflammatory diet must:

- Eliminate sugars and sweets, or include very little
- Only eat small amounts of meat: 3–6 oz. once or twice a day (3–4 oz. for women, 3–6 oz. for men)
- Limit red meat to 3–6 oz. once or twice a week, or eliminate completely
- Follow a mostly plant-based diet
- Eliminate or limit processed meats (hot dogs, salami, pepperoni, bacon, sausage, etc.)
- Include healthy starches with a low glycemic value, such as steel-cut oats, quinoa, beans, peas, lentils, sweet potatoes, etc.
- Avoid fried food
- Limit, avoid, or rotate every four days: pork, lamb, and shrimp, crab, lobster, or other shellfish
- Include healthy fats from macadamia nuts, cashews, walnuts, almonds, extra-virgin olive oil, and avocados
- Minimize intake of omega-6 fats (corn oil, safflower oil, sunflower oil, cottonseed oil, soybean oil)
- Include wild salmon (probably the highest anti-inflammatory food on the planet) and other wild, low-mercury fish
- Eliminate trans fats or hydrogenated fats
- Eliminate or limit grains (use legumes: beans, peas, lentils) or rotate every four days
- Reach a healthy body weight because obesity is connected to most diseases today
- Minimize night shades (peppers, tomatoes, potatoes, paprika, eggplant) or rotate every four days
- Be able to improve, or control, type 2 diabetes
- Include exercise five days a week and balance your hormones
- Cope with stress
- Include more sleep
- Eliminate or limit GMO foods (most soy, corn, canola oil, and cottonseed oil)

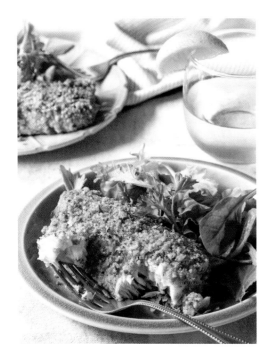

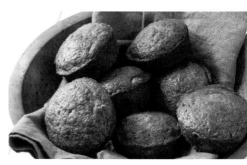

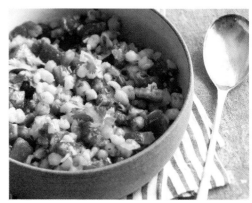

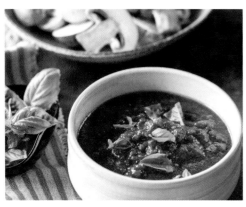

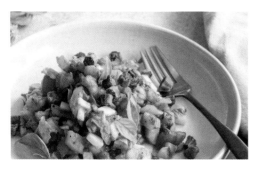

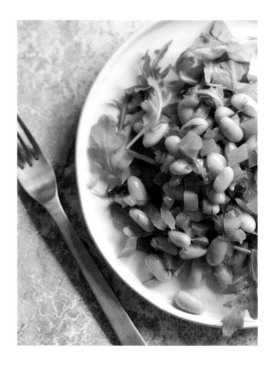

WEEK 2: DAY #8

BREAKFAST (6:00 A.M.):
- Smoothie made with 6 oz. plain coconut, almond, or skim milk, 1½ cups cubed, seedless watermelon, 1-2 tbsp. ground flaxseeds, 1 scoop plant protein powder, ½ banana (may add ice or sweeten with stevia to taste)
- 3 oz. turkey sausage (squeeze between two napkins to remove fat)
- Handful of walnuts (approximately 5-10)
- 1 cup of green tea or coffee, sweetened with stevia, coconut milk for creamer

MID-MORNING SNACK (9:00 A.M.):
- 1 banana

LUNCH (12:00 P.M.):
- Sliced chicken (3-4 oz. for women, 3-6 oz. for men) on a bed of chopped cabbage with shredded carrot (as much as desired)
- 1 cup tomato basil soup
- Large salad with artichoke hearts, red bell peppers, a small amount of grated Parmesan cheese, and extra-virgin olive oil and balsamic vinegar as dressing (no croutons)
- 1 cup of green tea, water, sparkling water, or unsweetened iced tea with lemon or lime

MID-AFTERNOON SNACK (3:00 P.M.):

- Handful of walnuts (approximately 5-10)

DINNER (6:00 P.M.):

- Extra lean beef (96/4, petite fillet) seasoned with black pepper (3-4 oz. for women, 3-6 oz. for men)
- Oven-roasted okra with a small amount of salt (as much as desired)
- ⅓ cup Tabbuouleh
- Large salad with plenty of colorful vegetables and extra-virgin olive oil and balsamic vinegar as dressing (no croutons)
- 1 cup of green tea, water, sparkling water, or unsweetened iced tea with lemon or lime

EVENING SNACK (9:00 P.M.):

- Broth-based vegetable soup without potatoes or pasta (½ cup for women, 1 cup for men)

FOOD FACT: EGGS

Sizes: Eggs are sold in six different sizes, ranging from jumbo to peewee. Sizing is based on the weight per dozen as the eggs are graded. For most recipes, large eggs are suggested.

Shells: The color of the eggshell is determined by the breed of the hen. The nutritional content and taste does not vary between colors of the shell. FYI: it takes twenty-six hours for a hen to produce an egg and twenty of those hours are spent forming the shell.

DAY #9

BREAKFAST (6:00 A.M.):
- Omelet (1 yolk, 3 whites) made with sliced mushrooms and chopped onion pieces cooked in a small amount of organic butter or extra-virgin olive oil
- 1 slice gluten-free bread, toasted
- ½ cup sliced strawberries
- 1 cup of green tea or coffee, sweetened with stevia, coconut milk for creamer

MID-MORNING SNACK (9:00 A.M.):
- ¼ cup blueberries

LUNCH (12:00 P.M.):
- Grilled turkey tenderloin with black and lemon pepper (3-4 oz. for women, 3-6 oz. for men)
- Gazpacho salad: Mix chopped cucumber, tomato and onion pieces with garlic and herbs. Combine with lemon juice, olive oil, red wine vinegar, and black pepper, and pour over a large amount of baby spinach leaves (no croutons)
- 1 cup of green tea, water, sparkling water, or unsweetened iced tea with lemon or lime

MID-AFTERNOON SNACK (3:00 P.M.):
- Handful of macadamia nuts (approximately 5-10)

DINNER (6:00 P.M.):

- Baked tilapia with citrus marinade and chopped fresh dill (3-6 oz. for women, 3-8 oz. for men)
- Steamed Swiss chard (as much as desired)
- Large salad with plenty of colorful vegetables and extra-virgin olive oil and balsamic vinegar as dressing (no croutons)
- 1 cup of green tea, water, sparkling water, or unsweetened iced tea with lemon or lime

EVENING SNACK (9:00 P.M.):

- Carrot sticks with ¼ cup edamame guacamole (puree shelled edamame with 1 avocado slice, 1 tsp. lemon juice, and 1 dash hot sauce)

FOOD FACTS: PECANS

Origin: Pecans are the only tree nuts that are native to North America. They are members of the hickory family.

Botany: Pecan trees can take up to twenty years to produce a full crop of nuts. There are more than five-hundred varieties of pecans that exist worldwide today, but only a few are produced on a wide commercial scale. The most popular varieties in the South are Cape Fear, Desirable, Elliott, and Schley.

Chopping: My favorite way to chop pecans is to put the amount I need in a sealed freezer bag. Then I just pull out my kitchen mallet and give it a few raps on the cutting board. The pecans are broken up and ready to use.

DAY #10

BREAKFAST (6:00 A.M.):
- 2 buck wheat pancakes with ½ cup blackberries sautéed in 1 pat of organic butter
- 3 oz. turkey bacon (squeeze between two napkins to remove fat)
- 1 cup of green tea or coffee, sweetened with stevia, coconut milk for creamer

MID-MORNING SNACK (9:00 A.M.):
- 1 nectarine or peach

LUNCH (12:00 P.M.):
- Grilled shrimp (large) kabob with spice rub (8 for women, 12 for men)
- Roasted eggplant (as much as desired) with fresh chopped oregano and black pepper
- 1 cup of green tea, water, sparkling water, or unsweetened iced tea with lemon or lime

MID-AFTERNOON SNACK (3:00 P.M.):
- Handful of pecans (approximately 5-10)

DINNER (6:00 P.M.):
- Broiled catfish filet (3-4 oz. for women, 3-6 oz. for men) with minced garlic, finely-chopped pecans, and cracked black pepper

- ½ cup mushroom and pearl barley stuffing
- Large salad with plenty of colorful vegetables and extra-virgin olive oil and balsamic vinegar as dressing (no croutons)
- 1 cup of green tea, water, sparkling water, or unsweetened iced tea with lemon or lime

EVENING SNACK (9:00 P.M.):

- 1 cup kale chips

FOOD FACTS: SHELLFISH

Soft-shell crabs are in season from April through about the third week of September, with peaks in June and July.

Crawfish are sometimes called crayfish or crawdads. Like lobster, they turn bright red when cooked. They typically range from 2-7 ounces.

The most popular shellfish in the United States is shrimp, followed by crab.

DAY #11

BREAKFAST (6:00 A.M.):

- Hash browns or sweet potato hash browns
  (½ cup for women, 1 cup for men) with diced
  onion pieces and cooked under low heat with
  olive oil
- 1 avocado, peeled, sliced, and sprinkled with
  1 tsp. lime juice
- ½ cup blueberries
- Handful of almonds (approximately 5-10)
- 1 cup of green tea or coffee, sweetened with stevia,
  coconut milk for creamer

MID-MORNING SNACK (9:00 A.M.):

- 1 plum or tangerine

LUNCH (12:00 P.M.):

- Black bean and crawfish (3-6 oz. for women,
  3-8 oz. for men) tacos with chopped tomato
  on gluten-free tortillas
- 1 cup white and black bean soup
- Large salad with radishes, carrots, shallots,
  and extra-virgin olive oil and balsamic vinegar
  as dressing (no croutons)
- 1 cup of green tea, water, sparkling water,
  or unsweetened iced tea with lemon or lime

MID-AFTERNOON SNACK (3:00 P.M.):

- Handful of almonds (approximately 5-10)

DINNER (6:00 P.M.):

- Grilled boneless, skinless chicken breast (3-4 oz. for women, 3-6 oz. for men) with chopped fresh basil and lemon juice
- Steamed broccoli (as much as desired) with black pepper and a small amount of salt
- Large salad with plenty of colorful vegetables and extra-virgin olive oil and balsamic vinegar as dressing (no croutons)
- 1 cup of green tea, water, sparkling water, or unsweetened iced tea with lemon or lime

EVENING SNACK (9:00 P.M.):

- Celery sticks and ¼ cup gluten-free almond butter

FOOD FACT: SWEET POTATOES

Storage: Sweet potatoes are really no different from regular potatoes as far as the best way to store them. Both excel in cool, dry, well-ventilated places. The ideal storage temperature is 55°F. When properly stored, you can easily keep sweet potatoes up to a month. Do not refrigerate raw potatoes, only cooked leftovers. Refrigerating them raw will cause a hard core to develop, as well as hasten decay.

DAY #12

BREAKFAST (6:00 A.M.):
- 2 slices of gluten-free French toast: for batter, mix together ¼ tsp. cinnamon, ¼ tsp. vanilla extract, 2-3 egg whites and 1 yolk, and dip both sides of bread in batter; top with ¼ cup berries (blackberries, strawberries, raspberries, or blueberries)
- Smoothie made with 6 oz. plain coconut, almond, or skim milk, ½ frozen banana or 1 tbsp. almond butter, ¼ cup frozen blueberries or raspberries, 1-2 tbsp. ground flaxseeds, 1 scoop plant protein powder (may add ice or sweeten with stevia to taste)
- 1 cup of green tea or coffee, sweetened with stevia, coconut milk for creamer

MID-MORNING SNACK (9:00 A.M.):
- ¼ cup strawberries

LUNCH (12:00 P.M.):
- Grilled wild salmon (3-6 oz. for women, 3-8 oz. for men) with lime juice and chopped cilantro
- Baked sweet potato (size of 1 tennis ball for women, size of 1-2 tennis ball(s) for men) with 1 pat of organic butter
- Large salad with arugula, white beans, orange bell pepper, and extra-virgin olive oil, lemon juice, and fresh dill as dressing (no croutons)
- 1 cup of green tea, water, sparkling water, or unsweetened iced tea with lemon or lime

MID-AFTERNOON SNACK (3:00 P.M.):

- ½ cup hummus with 1-2 slices gluten-free pita bread

DINNER (6:00 P.M.):

- Grilled chicken (3-4 oz. for women, 3-6 oz. for men) with marjoram
- 1 cup coleslaw: shred half a head of cabbage and mix with 1-2 tbsp. light mayonnaise, ½ cup apple cider vinegar, 1 tbsp. celery seed, and 1 grated carrot
- Broth-based vegetable soup without potatoes or pasta (½ cup for women, 1 cup for men)
- Large salad with plenty of colorful vegetables and extra-virgin olive oil and balsamic vinegar as dressing (no croutons)
- Steamed broccoli (as much as desired)
- 1 cup of green tea, water, sparkling water, or unsweetened iced tea with lemon or lime

EVENING SNACK (9:00 P.M.):

- Handful of cashews (approximately 5-10)

FOOD FACT: BROCCOLI

Selection: Keep in mind that broccoli is a flower that wants to bloom. But we don't want it to do so when we consume it. Look for tightly closed florets that are compact. Then, smell it, and you should notice a fresh aroma rather than something that smells cabbage-like.

DAY #13

BREAKFAST (6:00 A.M.):

- ½ broiled grapefruit sprinkled with ½ tsp. chia seeds
- 1-2 slices gluten-free bread, toasted and topped with sliced avocado
- Smoothie made with 6 oz. plain coconut, almond, or skim milk, 1 cup strawberries, 1 frozen banana, 1-2 tbsp. ground flaxseeds, 1 scoop plant protein powder (may add ice or sweeten with stevia to taste)
- 1 cup of green tea or coffee, sweetened with stevia, coconut milk for creamer

MID-MORNING SNACK (9:00 A.M.):

- ½ cup cubed pineapple or 1 fig

LUNCH (12:00 P.M.):

- Grilled chicken breast (3-4 oz. for women, 3-6 oz. for men) topped with sliced pineapple
- 1 cup broth-based minestrone soup or vegetable soup without potatoes or pasta
- Balsamic glazed zucchini (as much as desired), topped with fresh basil
- Large salad with mushrooms, green onions, bell peppers, and extra-virgin olive oil and balsamic vinegar as dressing (no croutons)
- 1 cup of green tea, water, sparkling water, or unsweetened iced tea with lemon or lime

MID-AFTERNOON SNACK (3:00 P.M.):

- Handful of pistachio nuts (approximately 5-10)

DINNER (6:00 P.M.):

- Grilled scallops (3-6 oz. for women, 3-8 oz. for men) with cremini mushroom kabob (6 mushrooms) brushed with 1 tbsp. olive oil and herbs de provence
- Steamed spinach with crushed red pepper and a small amount of grated Parmesan cheese (as much as desired)
- Large salad with plenty of colorful vegetables and extra-virgin olive oil and balsamic vinegar as dressing (no croutons)
- 1 cup of green tea, water, sparkling water, or unsweetened iced tea with lemon or lime

EVENING SNACK (9:00 P.M.):

- Minestrone soup with chickpeas (½ cup for women, 1 cup for men)

FOOD FACT: APPLES

Freezing: Crush a vitamin C tablet to make ½ teaspoon and stir into 1 quart of cold water. Wash, peel, core, and slice the apples. Use only firm slices for freezing. Dip the slice in the water and allow to soak for 1 minute. Remove and drain on paper towels. Transfer to a baking sheet in a single layer and place in the freezer. When frozen solid, place in a freezer container, label, date, and keep in freezer.

DAY #14

BREAKFAST (6:00 A.M.):
- 1 gluten-free bagel, toasted, spread with 1 pat of organic butter, and topped with 1 tbsp. toasted, unsalted sunflower seeds
- 1 banana
- 1 cup plain, gluten-free Greek yogurt
- 1 cup of green tea or coffee, sweetened with stevia, coconut milk for creamer

MID-MORNING SNACK (9:00 A.M.):
- 1 Granny Smith apple

LUNCH (12:00 P.M.):
- Veggie burger patty (no bun) topped with arugula, sliced tomato, and sprinkled with chives (3-4 oz. for women, 3-6 oz. for men)
- Baked sweet potato (size of 1 tennis ball for women, size of 1-2 tennis ball(s) for men) with 1 pat of organic butter
- Carrot salad with golden raisins, manadrin oranges, pitted black olives, topped with cashews
- 1 cup of green tea, water, sparkling water, or unsweetened iced tea with lemon or lime

MID-AFTERNOON SNACK (3:00 P.M.):
- Handful of unsalted, roasted peanuts (approximately 5-10)

DINNER (6:00 P.M.):

- Grilled tropical chicken kabobs with fresh pineapple and onion (3-4 oz. for women, 3-6 oz. for men)
- Roasted beets or Brussels sprouts (as much as desired) with minced garlic and black pepper
- Steamed cauliflower (as much as desired)
- Large salad with plenty of colorful vegetables and extra-virgin olive oil and balsamic vinegar as dressing (no croutons)
- 1 cup of green tea, water, sparkling water, or unsweetened iced tea with lemon or lime

EVENING SNACK (9:00 P.M.):

- Celery sticks with ¼ cup gluten-free peanut butter spread

FOOD FACT: GROUND MEAT

Selection: Ground meats are sold according to the proportion of fat to lean. When you see a label that says 80/20, that means it has 20 percent fat and the rest is lean. Always look for those with the lowest fat content, such as 90/10. But remember that fat is what makes the meat brown nicely, so when cooked, it will not have a characteristic brown color as those with a higher fat content.

GLUTEN IS EVERYWHERE

According to the Celiac Disease Foundation (celiac.org), there are many sources of gluten. The following grains and their derivatives are sources of gluten:

- Wheat; varieties and derivatives of wheat such as:
  wheat berries, durum, emmer, semolina, spelt, farina, faro, graham, KAMUT°
  khorasan wheat, einkorn wheat
- Rye
- Barley
- Triticale
- Malt in various forms including: malted barley flour, malted milk or milk shakes, malt extract, malt syrup, malt flavoring, malt vinegar
- Brewer's yeast
- Wheat starch that has not been processed to remove the presence of gluten to below 20 parts per million and adhere to the FDA labeling law

Common foods that contain gluten:

- Pastas: raviolis, dumplings, couscous, and gnocchi
- Noodles: ramen, udon, soba (those made with only a percentage of buckwheat flour), chow mein, and egg noodles (Note: rice noodles and mung bean noodles are gluten free)
- Breads and pastries: croissants, pita, naan, bagels, flatbreads, corn bread, potato bread, muffins, donuts, rolls
- Crackers: pretzels, Goldfish crackers, graham crackers
- Baked goods: cakes, cookies, pie crusts, brownies
- Cereal and granola: corn flakes and rice puffs often contain malt extract/flavoring, granola is often made with regular oats not gluten-free oats
- Breakfast foods: pancakes, waffles, French toast, crepes, biscuits
- Breading and coating mixes: panko bread crumbs
- Croutons: stuffings, dressings
- Sauces and gravies (many use wheat flour as a thickener): traditional soy sauce, cream sauces made with a roux
- Flour tortillas
- Beer (unless explicitly gluten-free) and any malt beverages
- Brewer's yeast
- Anything else that uses "wheat flour" as an ingredient

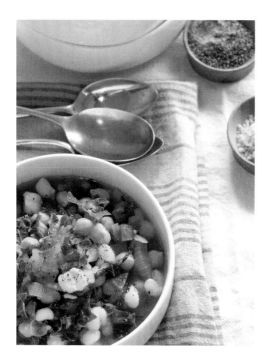

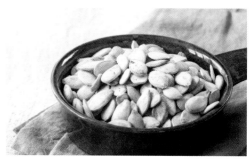

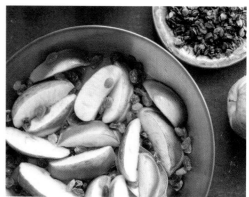

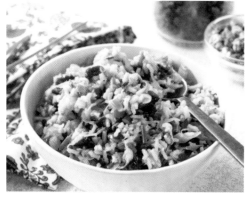

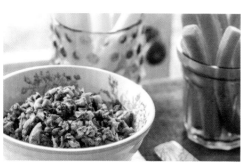

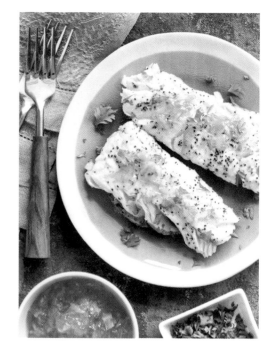

WEEK 3: DAY #15

BREAKFAST (6:00 A.M.):

- ½ cup gluten-free natural granola (no sugar)
- 2 (6-7 inch) mixed fruit kabobs (assemble with equal amounts of cubed melons, strawberries, and grapes)
- Smoothie made with 6 oz. plain coconut, almond, or skim milk, ½ cup frozen blueberries, 1 scoop plant protein powder, 1-2 tbsp. ground flaxseeds (may add ice or sweeten with stevia to taste)
- 1 cup of green tea or coffee, sweetened with stevia, coconut milk for creamer

MID-MORNING SNACK (9:00 A.M.):

- ¼ cup blackberries

LUNCH (12:00 P.M.):

- Extra lean beef (96/4, petite fillet) seasoned with black pepper (3-4 oz. for women, 3-6 oz. for men)
- Broth-based vegetable soup without potatoes or pasta (½ cup for women, 1 cup for men)
- Four bean salad with kindey, white, black, and garbanzo beans, topped with chopped green bell pepper and shallots, and apple cider vinegar, extra-virgin olive oil, basil, and tarragon as dressing
- 1 cup of green tea, water, sparkling water, or unsweetened iced tea with lemon or lime

MID-AFTERNOON SNACK (3:00 P.M.):

- Handful of walnuts (approximately 5-10)

DINNER (6:00 P.M.):

- Ground turkey burger (no bun) topped with cumin and a small amount of crumbled Feta (3-4 oz. for women, 3-6 oz. for men)
- Celery sticks with ¼ cup pineapple salsa
- Steamed turnip greens or bok choy (as much as desired)
- Large salad with plenty of colorful vegetables and extra-virgin olive oil and balsamic vinegar as dressing (no croutons)
- 1 cup of green tea, water, sparkling water, or unsweetened iced tea with lemon or lime

EVENING SNACK (9:00 P.M.):

- Stewed apples topped with rolled oats and 1 tbsp. of Greek yogurt

FOOD FACTS: GREENS

Selection: Greens should be green! Avoid purchasing any that show signs of yellowing or wilting, which are indicators of old age.

Storage: Keep greens in the crisper drawer or the bottom of your refrigerator. They like high humidity, so sprinkle the bag with a bit of water in case you won't be using them right away. For best quality, use within 2 days.

DAY #16

BREAKFAST (6:00 A.M.):
- ¾ cup gluten-free, high-fiber cinnamon cereal with 8 oz. coconut, almond, or skim milk and ¼ cup blueberries
- 1 banana
- Handful of macadamia nuts (approximately 5-10)
- 1 cup of green tea or coffee, sweetened with stevia, coconut milk for creamer

MID-MORNING SNACK (9:00 A.M.):
- 1 pear (cored and peeled) or ½ pomegranate

LUNCH (12:00 P.M.):
- Rosemary-rubbed, baked boneless, skinless chicken breast (3-4 oz. for women, 3-6 oz. for men)
- ¼ cup Northern or white bean dip (puree leftovers from previous day's lunch, topped with lemon juice and black pepper) with gluten-free, toasted pita triangles
- Large salad with sliced zucchini and radishes, chopped shallot pieces, snow peas, and extra-virgin olive oil and balsamic vinegar as dressing (no croutons)
- 1 cup of green tea, water, sparkling water, or unsweetened iced tea with lemon or lime

MID-AFTERNOON SNACK (3:00 P.M.):
- Handful of macadamia nuts (approximately 5-10)

DINNER (6:00 P.M.):

- Pan-blackened snapper
  (3-6 oz. for women, 3-8 oz. for men)
- Steamed green beans with chopped tomatoes, garlic, and pearl onions (as much as desired)
- Large salad with plenty of colorful vegetables and extra-virgin olive oil and balsamic vinegar as dressing (no croutons)
- 1 cup of green tea, water, sparkling water, or unsweetened iced tea with lemon or lime

EVENING SNACK (9:00 P.M.):

- 1 cup kale chips

FOOD FACTS: ONIONS

Storage: Fresh onions, like green onions, should always be stored in the refrigerator. Bulb onions can be stored at room temperature, but the shelf life is extended greatly if you have room in the refrigerator.

Aroma: The distinct smell of onions is terrific, but you don't want it to transfer to your more odor-sensitive items that might be close by. For that reason, make sure they are placed in loosely closed plastic bags and, if possible, in a different crisper drawer from fruits.

DAY #17

BREAKFAST (6:00 A.M.):
- Omelet (1 yolk, 3 whites) made with sliced mushrooms and chopped onion cooked in a small amount of organic butter or extra-virgin olive oil
- 1 slice gluten-free bread, toasted
- ½ cup blueberries
- 1 cup of green tea or coffee, sweetened with stevia, coconut milk for creamer

MID-MORNING SNACK (9:00 A.M.):
- 1 clementine or tangerine

LUNCH (12:00 P.M.):
- Fresh Fish tacos (one fish filet for three tacos)
- 2 leek and wilted kale stuffed portabella mushrooms
- Large salad with jicama, tomatoes, carrots, and extra-virgin olive oil and balsamic vinegar as dressing (no croutons)
- 1 cup of green tea, water, sparkling water, or unsweetened iced tea with lemon or lime

MID-AFTERNOON SNACK (3:00 P.M.):
- Handful of pecans (approximately 5-10)

DINNER (6:00 P.M.):

- Baked wild salmon with fresh dill
  (3-6 oz. for women, 3-8 oz. for men)
- Roasted patty pan, acorn, zucchini, or yellow
  squash with fresh chopped oregano or thyme
  (as much as desired)
- Steamed asparagus (as much as desired)
- Large salad with plenty of colorful vegetables
  and extra-virgin olive oil and balsamic vinegar
  as dressing (no croutons)
- 1 cup of green tea, water, sparkling water,
  or unsweetened iced tea with lemon or lime

EVENING SNACK (9:00 P.M.):

- 1 lettuce wrap with asparagus and chicken

FOOD FACT: MANGO

Selection: Use your nose to select a good mango. If there isn't a faintly-sweet aroma around the stem, chances are it doesn't have any flavor. Choose firm fruit with a tight skin and nothing that looks wrinkled or loose.

DAY #18

BREAKFAST (6:00 A.M.):
- ½ cup gluten-free natural granola with 1 tbsp. roasted pumpkin seeds
- ½ broiled grapefruit sprinkled with ½ tsp. chia seeds
- Smoothie made with 6 oz. plain coconut, almond, or skim milk, 1 cup frozen papayas or mangos, 1-2 tbsp. ground flaxseeds (may add ice or sweeten with stevia to taste)
- 1 cup of green tea or coffee, sweetened with stevia, coconut milk for creamer

MID-MORNING SNACK (9:00 A.M.):
- ¼ cup strawberries

LUNCH (12:00 P.M.):
- Sliced turkey (3-4 oz. for women, 3-6 oz. for men), 1 thinly sliced, peeled apple and spinach on gluten-free pita bread
- Steamed carrots (as much as desired) with drizzle from squeezed half of a fresh orange
- Large salad with broccoli slaw and extra-virgin olive oil and balsamic vinegar as dressing (no croutons)
- 1 cup of green tea, water, sparkling water, or unsweetened iced tea with lemon or lime

MID-AFTERNOON SNACK (3:00 P.M.):
- 1 tbsp. of roasted pumpkin seeds

DINNER (6:00 P.M.):

- Pan-roasted whitefish (3-6 oz. for women, 3-8 oz. for men) with citrus juice and parsley
- Broiled eggplant with chopped fresh oregano
- Herbed broiled mushrooms with chopped fresh parsley and chives
- Large salad with plenty of colorful vegetables and extra-virgin olive oil and balsamic vinegar as dressing (no croutons)
- 1 cup of green tea, water, sparkling water, or unsweetened iced tea with lemon or lime

EVENING SNACK (9:00 P.M.):

- 6 whole, raw mushrooms and 4 carrot sticks

FOOD FACTS: ASPARAGUS

Selection: The important thing is to choose an asparagus bunch with spears that are very close in diameter to one another. This translates into even cooking.

Storage: Store asparagus unwashed and untrimmed in a plastic bag in the refrigerator crisper drawer. It will keep up to 3 days, but the sooner you use it, the better it will taste. Trim or snap off the hard, fibrous, white bottoms before use. It is not necessary to peel the scales off asparagus before use, but if you do, use a paring knife or vegetable peeler to get the job done.

DAY #19

BREAKFAST (6:00 A.M.):
- Steel-cut oatmeal cooked with ground cinnamon and ¼ cup blueberries
- 2-3 oz. turkey bacon or turkey sausage (squeeze between two napkins to remove fat)
- Handful of pecans (approximately 5-10)
- 1 cup of green tea or coffee, sweetened with stevia, coconut milk for creamer

MID-MORNING SNACK (9:00 A.M.):
- 1 tangerine or navel orange

LUNCH (12:00 P.M.):
- Tuna wrap: tongol tuna (3-6 oz. for women, 3-8 oz. for men) with 1 tbsp. light mayonnaise, sliced tomato, and romaine lettuce on 1-2 slices brown rice bread or gluten-free bread
- 1 cup lima beans
- Large salad with mushrooms, bell peppers, carrots, tomatoes, and extra-virgin olive oil and balsamic vinegar as dressing (no croutons)
- 1 cup of green tea, water, sparkling water, or unsweetened iced tea with lemon or lime

MID-AFTERNOON SNACK (3:00 P.M.):
- 1 tbsp. of roasted sunflower or pumpkin seeds

DINNER (6:00 P.M.):

- Roasted turkey breast
  (3-4 oz. for women, 3-6 oz. for men)
- Steamed green beans (as much as desired) seasoned
  with lemon pepper, garlic, or a small amount of salt
- Large salad with plenty of colorful vegetables
  and extra-virgin olive oil and balsamic vinegar
  as dressing (no croutons)
- 1 cup of green tea, water, sparkling water,
  or unsweetened iced tea with lemon or lime

EVENING SNACK (9:00 P.M.):

- Broth-based vegetable soup without potatoes or
  pasta (½ cup for women, 1 cup for men)

FOOD FACTS: OKRA

Selection: The smaller the better, so look for pods that are less than six inches long. Larger, older ones tend to be quite tough and fibrous.

Freezing: I like to freeze excess okra whole but it is necessary to blanch it first. Start by bringing a large pot of water to a boil. Meanwhile, trim the stem ends of the okra pods, being careful not to expose the seed cell. Plunge into the boiling water for three minutes, then plunge into ice-cold water for three minutes. Drain well on paper towels before packing into freezer containers. Make sure you label and date the package before freezing.

DAY #20

BREAKFAST (6:00 A.M.):
- 2 buck wheat pancakes with ½ cup chopped papayas or mangos
- Handful of pistachio nuts (approximately 5-10)
- 1 cup of green tea or coffee, sweetened with stevia, coconut milk for creamer

MID-MORNING SNACK (9:00 A.M.):
- 1 kiwi, peeled and sliced

LUNCH (12:00 P.M.):
- Turkey salad mixed with black pepper and 1 tbsp. light mayonnaise on gluten-free toasted bread (3-4 oz. for women, 3-6 oz. for men)
- Roasted okra (as much as desired)
- Large salad with cucumbers, corn, red bell pepper, onion, and extra-virgin olive oil and balsamic vinegar as dressing (no croutons)
- 1 cup of green tea, water, sparkling water, or unsweetened iced tea with lemon or lime

MID-AFTERNOON SNACK (3:00 P.M.):
- Handful of pistachio nuts (approximately 5-10)

DINNER (6:00 P.M.):

- Broiled freshwater trout (3-6 oz. for women, 3-8 oz. for men) topped with ¼ cup tomatillo or tomato salsa
- ½ cup brown rice and berry pilaf, topped with chopped walnuts
- Large salad with plenty of colorful vegetables and extra-virgin olive oil and balsamic vinegar as dressing (no croutons)
- 1 cup of green tea, water, sparkling water, or unsweetened iced tea with lemon or lime

EVENING SNACK (9:00 P.M.):

- Baked tortilla chips with ¼ cup fresh tomato salsa

FOOD FACTS: TOMATOES

Keep bruises at bay: On the market, tomatoes are displayed with the bottoms up in order to make selection easier and for it to look nicer. Don't copy this at home. Tomatoes should be stored as they grow on the vine, with the stem end up. Why? The most delicate part of the tomato is the easily bruised shoulders around the stem.

DAY #21

BREAKFAST (6:00 A.M.):

- 1 gluten-free bagel, toasted with a smear of organic butter and 1 tsp. slivered almonds
- ½ broiled grapefruit sprinkled with ½ tsp. chia seeds
- 1 cup gluten-free plain, Greek yogurt
- 1 cup of green tea or coffee, sweetened with stevia, coconut milk for creamer

MID-MORNING SNACK (9:00 A.M.):

- ½ cup seedless grapes

LUNCH (12:00 P.M.):

- Roast beef and quinoa wraps (3-4 oz. for women, 3-6 oz. for men) wrapped in gluten-free tortillas
- 1 cup black beans with chopped celery and diced onion pieces
- Large salad with tomatoes, jicama, mushrooms, and extra-virgin olive oil and balsamic vinegar as dressing (no croutons)
- 1 cup of green tea, water, sparkling water, or unsweetened iced tea with lemon or lime

MID-AFTERNOON SNACK (3:00 P.M.):

- Handful of almonds (approximately 5-10)

DINNER (6:00 P.M.):

- Extra lean beef (96/4, petite fillet) seasoned with black pepper (3-4 oz. for women, 3-6 oz. for men)
- Grilled cremini mushrooms (as much as desired) on rosemary skewers with 1 tbsp. olive oil drizzle
- Large salad with plenty of colorful vegetables and extra-virgin olive oil and balsamic vinegar as dressing (no croutons)
- 1 cup of green tea, water, sparkling water, or unsweetened iced tea with lemon or lime

EVENING SNACK (9:00 P.M.):

- 1 lettuce wrap with roasted cauliflower and onion

FOOD FACT: MUSHROOMS

Storage: The main causes of decay in mushrooms are warm air and water, so keep them cool and dry. That means you shouldn't wash them until just before use.

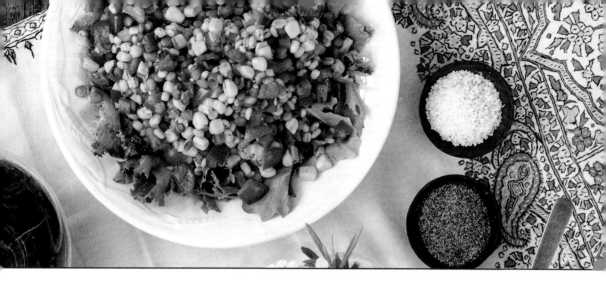

RECIPES

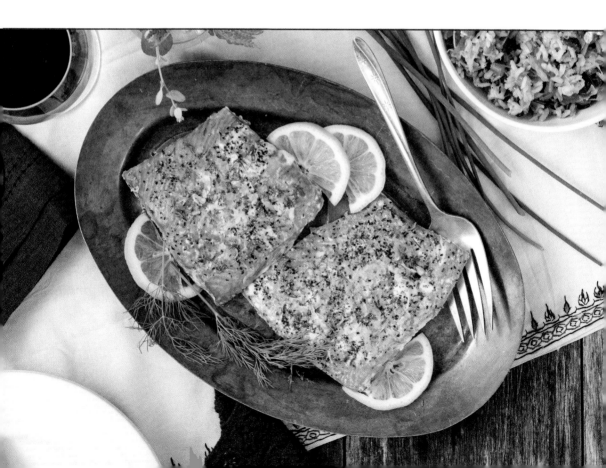

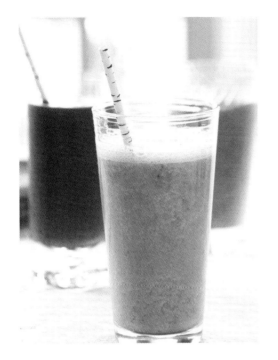

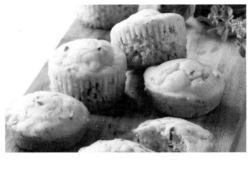

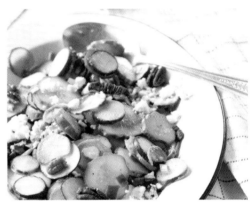

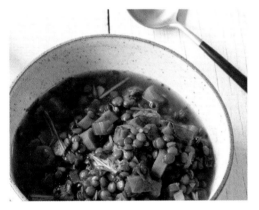

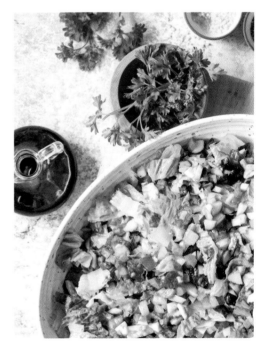

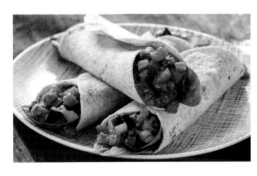

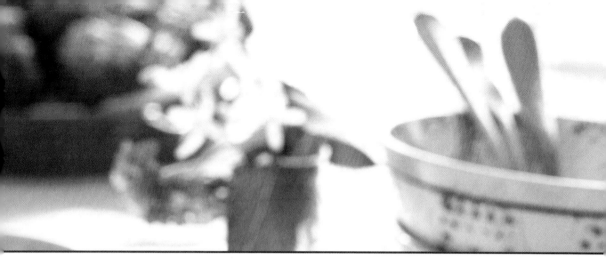

WEEK ONE

Days 1–7

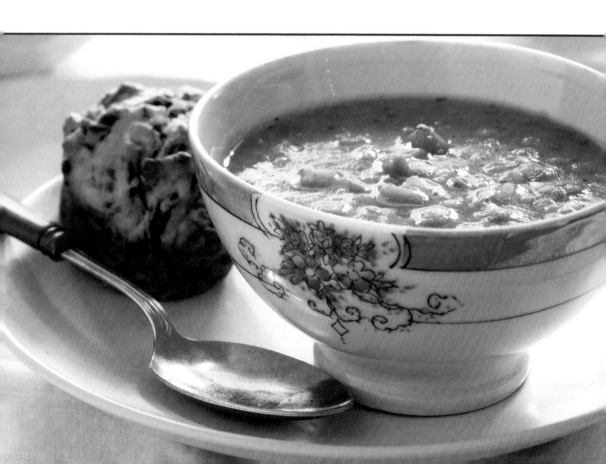

SHOBPING LIST – WEEK 1

(DAYS 1–7)

FRUITS

- ☐ Apricot – 1
- ☐ Bananas – 4
- ☐ Blueberries – 6-ounce package
- ☐ Cantaloupe or Honeydew – 1
- ☐ Grapefruit – 1 small
- ☐ Kiwi – 1
- ☐ Pear – 1
- ☐ Raspberries – 6 ounce package
- ☐ Seedless Grapes or Cherries
  – 1 small bag
- ☐ Strawberries – 16-ounce package
- ☐ Watermelon – 1 small

VEGETABLES

- ☐ Asparagus – 3 bunches
- ☐ Avocadoes – 3
- ☐ Bean Sprouts – 4-ounce package
- ☐ Broccoli – 7 day supply
- ☐ Cabbage – 1 head
- ☐ Cauliflower – 2 heads
- ☐ Corn – 1 ear
- ☐ Cucumbers – 7 day supply
- ☐ Eggplant – 2
- ☐ English Peas – 1 serving size
- ☐ Green Beans – 7 day supply
- ☐ Kale – 7 day supply
- ☐ Mushrooms – 7 day supply
- ☐ Peppers (variety of colors)
  – 7 day supply

- ☐ Pimentos – 1 small jar
- ☐ Salad Greens (chicory, spinach, kale, Belgian endive, bean sprouts, iceberg, romaine) – 7 day supply for twice daily salads
- ☐ Spaghetti Squash – 1 small
- ☐ Summer (Yellow, Zucchini) or Winter (Acorn, Butternut) Squash – 7 day supply
- ☐ Tomatoes – 7 day supply
- ☐ Zucchini – 4 medium size

MEAT

- ☐ Boneless, Skinless Chicken Breast – 2*
- ☐ Crab Meat*
- ☐ Extra Lean Beef (96/4, petite fillet)*
- ☐ Flounder*
- ☐ Mackerel*
- ☐ Salmon Fillet*
- ☐ Shrimp (large)*
- ☐ Turkey Breast Tenderloin – 4*
- ☐ Whitefish Fillet*

amount varies by gender
(see meal plan)

MERCURY IN FISH

The amount of mercury in fish depends on factors such as the type of fish, what it eats, and where it lives. According to the Natural Resources Defense Council, this is the recommendation for eating fish:

- **Fish with least mercury** *(eat freely)*: anchovies, butterfish, catfish, clams, crab (domestic), crawfish/crayfish, croaker (Atlantic), flounder, haddock (Atlantic), hake, herring, mackerel (N. Atlantic, chub), mullet, oyster, perch (ocean), plaice, pollock, salmon (canned or fresh), sardine, scallop, shad (American), shrimp, sole (Pacific), squid (calamari), tilapia, trout (freshwater), whitefish, and whiting

- **Fish with moderate mercury** *(eat six servings or less per month)*: bass (striped, black), carp, cod (Alaskan), croaker (white, Pacific), halibut (Atlantic, Pacific), jacksmelt, silverside, lobster, mahi mahi, monkfish, perch (freshwater), sablefish, skate, snapper, tuna (canned chunk light, skipjack), and weakfish (sea trout)

- **Fish with high mercury** *(eat three servings or less per month)*: bluefish, grouper, mackerel (Spanish, Gulf), sea bass (Chilean), and tuna (canned albacore, yellow fin)

- **Fish with highest mercury** *(avoid eating)*: mackerel (king), marlin, orange roughy, shark, swordfish, tilefish, and tuna (bigeye, ahi)

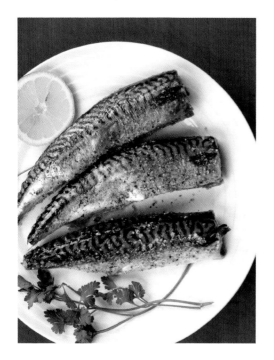

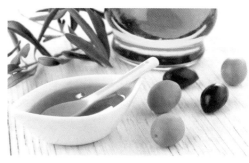

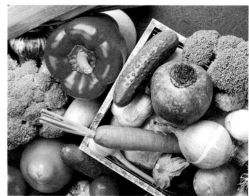

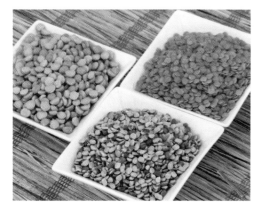

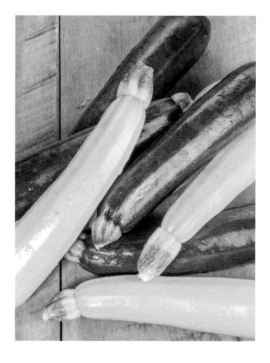

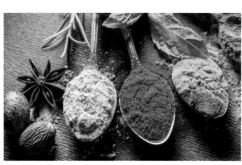

DAY 1

GRILLED TURKEY TENDERLOINS
Yield: 6 to 8 servings

Turkey tenderloins are great options for those who don't like to waste food. They come in a package of two, so this allows you to cook once and have plenty to stockpile in your freezer for later. If you don't want to grill the tenderloins, there's an option for roasting them in the oven.

1 (1¼ pound) package turkey
    tenderloins
1 tablespoon extra-virgin oil
1 tablespoon balsamic vinegar
1 tablespoon Dijon mustard
½ teaspoon garlic salt
¼ teaspoon black pepper
¼ teaspoon paprika

1. Place the turkey tenderloins in a large zip-top bag.
2. In a small bowl, whisk together the oil, vinegar, mustard, salt, pepper, and paprika.
3. Pour mixture over the turkey, seal the bag and gently massage to evenly coat. Refrigerate for up to 8 hours.
4. Remove the turkey from the refrigerator 20 minutes before grilling.

5. Preheat the grill to medium. Place the tenderloins on the rack and grill for 5 minutes.
6. Turn and grill for 5 minutes longer, basting with any sauce remaining in the bag.
7. Turn again and cook an additional 4 to 5 minutes or until an instant-read thermometer registers 165 degrees.
8. Remove from the grill and wrap in parchment paper to make a packet. Allow to rest 5 minutes before slicing and serving warm.

Option #2 (Roasting):
1. Preheat the oven to 350 degrees and lightly grease a baking dish.
2. Add the tenderloins and cover with aluminum foil.
3. Roast for 35 minutes. Remove from the oven and uncover.
4. Preheat the broiler to high.
5. Broil for 2 to 3 minutes until golden brown.
6. Cover with aluminum foil and allow to rest 5 minutes before slicing and serving warm.

GRILLED MACKEREL WITH FRESH TARRAGON
Yield: 2 servings

The firm flesh of mackerel means that the fillets can be grilled nicely without fear of them falling apart. The anise-like flavor of the perennial tarragon is a great match, but don't get carried away because the taste can quickly become overpowering.

2 mackerel fillets
1 tablespoon extra-virgin oil
½ teaspoon salt
¼ teaspoon dried tarragon
¼ teaspoon black pepper

1. Preheat the grill to medium-high.
2. Meanwhile, rub the mackerel on both sides with the oil.
3. Sprinkle evenly with the salt, tarragon, and pepper on the skinless side.
4. Grill with the skin side down for 3 minutes or until the skin is crispy.
5. Turn and grill another 2 minutes or until the fish is easily flaked with a fork. Serve warm.

EASY ROASTED VEGETABLES
Yield: 2 servings

This recipe will likely become a weekly regular for you, and it can transition from season to season to match produce availability. Just remember that the smaller the cut of the item, the shorter the roasting time. You will need to turn larger pieces of produce to make sure it is evenly roasted. Use a baking sheet with sides to catch any juices created as the vegetables roast.

3-4 cups vegetables (cauliflower, summer or winter squash, okra, sweet potatoes, carrots, beets, asparagus, mushrooms, parsnips, rutabagas, turnips, etc.)
1 teaspoon extra-virgin oil
½ teaspoon salt
¼ teaspoon black pepper

1. Preheat the oven to 350 degrees.
2. Lightly grease a baking sheet with sides with cooking spray.
3. Coarsely chop or slice the selected vegetables as desired and spread in a single layer on the baking sheet.
4. Drizzle with the oil and sprinkle evenly with the salt and pepper.
5. Roast for 20 to 30 minutes, turning larger pieces halfway through. Serve warm.

FOOD FACT: SQUASH (SUMMER)

Storage: Refrigeration is the key to extending the shelf life of any type of summer squash. Place it in the crisper drawer in an unclosed plastic bag.

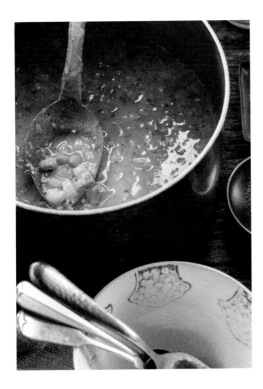

1 cup green split peas

1 cup yellow split peas

7 cups low sodium, organic vegetable or chicken stock (see page 96 or 117)

1 bay leaf

½ teaspoon dried thyme

½ teaspoon dried parsley

½ teaspoon dried chives

½ teaspoon seasoned salt

¼ teaspoon black pepper

Chopped fresh parsley for garnish

1. Place the oil in a Dutch oven over medium heat.
2. When hot, add the chopped onion pieces, carrots, celery, and garlic.
3. Sauté 3 minutes.
4. Add the green split peas, yellow split peas, stock, bay leaf, thyme, parsley, chives, salt, and pepper.
5. Bring to a boil, cover, and reduce the heat to low.
6. Simmer 2 hours. Remove from the heat and discard the bay leaf.
7. Serve warm with a garnish of fresh parsley.

LUSCIOUS SPLIT PEA SOUP
Yield: 6 servings

You might want to go ahead and mark this page because it's a recipe you'll likely return to again and again. While shopping for this recipe, look for both traditional green as well as yellow split peas at the supermarket to add visual interest to this soup.

1 tablespoon extra-virgin oil

1 large sweet onion, peeled and chopped

3 large carrots, peeled and chopped

3 celery stalks, chopped

3 garlic cloves, peeled and minced

FOOD FACT: CARROTS

Storage: As soon as I get them home, the tops come off. Then the delicious roots go into the crisper drawer, where they can reside for up to 2 weeks.

OLD-FASHIONED VEGETABLE SOUP
Yield: 6 servings

What could be more satisfying to the soul than a bowl of delicious vegetable soup? It is loaded with numerous nutrients all in one bowl. Go ahead and make this recipe over a weekend. You can enjoy it immediately, then later in the week, and you will still have enough to freeze for later use.

- 2 teaspoons extra-virgin oil
- 1 large sweet onion, peeled and chopped
- 3 garlic cloves, peeled and minced
- 3 carrots, peeled and chopped
- 2 celery stalks, chopped
- ½ parsnip, peeled and chopped
- 6 cups low sodium vegetable stock (see page 96)
- 1 yellow bell pepper, seeded and chopped
- 1 cup snapped green beans
- 2 large tomatoes, peeled and chopped
- 1 (14-ounce) can Northern or white beans, drained and rinsed
- ½ teaspoon dried basil
- ½ teaspoon dried oregano
- ½ teaspoon dried parsley
- ½ teaspoon seasoned salt
- ½ teaspoon crushed red pepper
- ¼ teaspoon black pepper
- Chopped fresh parsley for garnish

1. Place the oil in a Dutch oven over medium-high heat.
2. When hot, add the chopped onion pieces, garlic, carrots, celery, and parsnips.
3. Sauté for 4 minutes.
4. Add the stock, chopped bell pepper pieces, green beans, tomatoes, beans, basil, oregano, parsley, salt, red and black pepper.
5. Bring to a boil, cover, and reduce the heat to low.
6. Simmer for 1 hour or until the vegetables are tender. Serve warm.

STEAMED VEGETABLES
Yield: 2 servings

If you really want to preserve the nutrients in vegetables, steaming is better than boiling. A bonus is that no fat is necessary and it's quick.

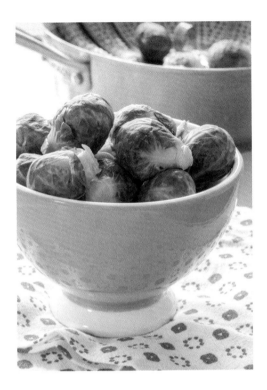

Caution: Remember that steam coming off the water is very hot, so always open the pan away from your face and use an oven mitt to avoid any burns.

Note: Don't overcrowd the basket. If you are steaming a very large amount, steam in batches to make sure the vegetables cook evenly.

3-4 cups vegetables of your choice, washed and cut in equal sizes

1. Bring a covered Dutch oven with at least 2 inches of water to a boil over medium-high heat.
2. Place the vegetables in the steamer basket.
3. If desired, place a few small sprigs of fresh herbs in the water, such as thyme or rosemary.
4. Reduce the heat to low and insert the steamer basket. Cover and simmer according to the guide here or until the vegetables are easily pierced with a paring knife in the thickest part. Drain and serve warm.

VEGETABLE STEAMING TIMES

Asparagus spears	3-5 minutes
Baby carrots	10-12 minutes
Broccoli florets	4-5 minutes
Broccoli spears	5-7 minutes
Brussels sprouts	8-9 minutes
Carrots, sliced	7-8 minutes
Cauliflower	7-9 minutes
English peas	3-5 minutes
Green beans	8 minutes
Kale, trimmed	4-7 minutes
Squash, summer	4-5 minutes
Squash, winter	15-20 minutes
Sweet potato cubes	20 minutes

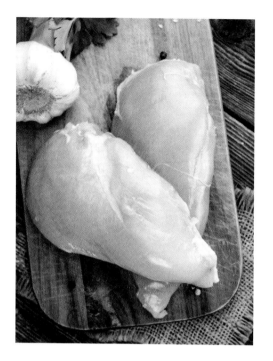

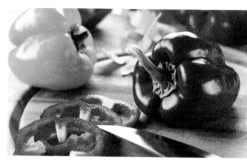

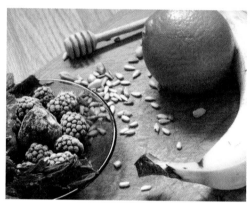

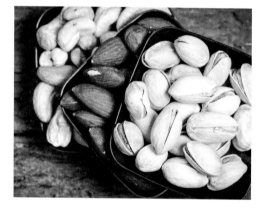

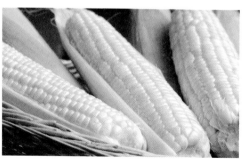

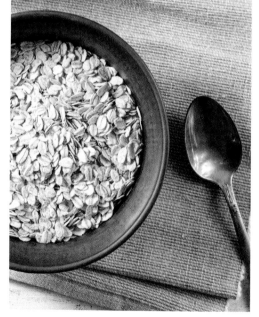

DAY 2

SLOW OATS
Yield: 3 to 4 servings

When using a slow cooker, it's always important to plan ahead. After a good night's rest, you want your food ready to eat. You will love this warm morning treat. Not only is it delicious, but the aroma is intoxicating! Add any fresh fruit you desire when serving, such as blueberries, sliced strawberries, or peaches.

1¼ cups old-fashioned oats
3 cups light, low sugar coconut milk (or
    can substitute 3 cups almond milk)
¾ cup water
1 banana, sliced
1-2 teaspoons organic stevia
1 teaspoon pure almond extract
1 teaspoon ground cinnamon
½ teaspoon ground ginger
⅛ teaspoon salt
Slivered toasted almonds for garnish

1. In a medium slow cooker, combine the oats, coconut milk, almond milk, water, bananas, brown sugar, extract, cinnamon, ginger, and salt.
2. Cover and cook on low for 8 hours.
3. Serve warm with a garnish of slivered almonds and/or fresh fruit.

ROASTED NUTS
Yield: 1 cup

The addition of heat to nuts of any kind greatly intensifies their flavor by bringing the essential oils to the surface. You will feel more satiated than if you ate the same amount plain!

1 cup whole nuts (pecans, walnuts,
    almonds, peanuts, pine nuts, etc.)

1. Preheat the oven to 350 degrees.
2. Meanwhile, spread the nuts in a single layer on a dry baking sheet.
3. Place in the preheated oven and roast for 5-6 minutes (smaller pieces roast for the shortest amount of time).
4. Shake the pan occasionally to toast all sides of the nuts evenly.
5. Remove from the oven and cool completely.

FOOD FACT: PECANS

Storage: Pecans can be placed in the freezer and should be used within one year, or you can store them in the refrigerator for up to six months.

FOOD FACT: BANANAS

Storage: Room temperature storage is best. The peel turns from green to yellow to yellow with brown dots. You can store overripe ones in the refrigerator. The outer peel will darken, but the flesh will be fine.

BREAKFAST FRUIT SMOOTHIES
Yield: 1 serving

These smoothies are a great nutritional start to your day. Include fruit options that are from your freezer, countertop, and refrigerator. If you don't include any frozen fruit, you might want to include some ice cubes to make sure it is frosty cold.

Option #1:
    ½ frozen banana
    ¼ cup frozen raspberries, blackberries, blueberries, or chopped strawberries
    1-2 tablespoons ground flaxseeds or chia seeds
    1 scoop plant protein powder
    1 tablespoon cashew nut or almond butter
    6 ounces coconut, almond, or skim milk
    If desired, you may add ice or sweeten with stevia to taste.

1. Process in a blender until smooth and serve immediately.

Option #2:
    1½ cups cubed frozen, seedless watermelon
    ½ frozen banana
    1-2 tablespoons ground flaxseeds or chia seeds
    1 scoop plant protein powder
    6 ounces coconut, almond, or skim milk
    If desired, you may add ice or sweeten with stevia to taste.

1. Process in a blender until smooth and serve immediately.

Option #3:
    ½ cup frozen blueberries, raspberries, or peaches
    ½ frozen banana
    1 tablespoon almond butter
    1-2 tablespoons ground flaxseeds or chia seeds
    1 scoop plant protein powder
    6 ounces coconut, almond, or skim milk
    If desired, you may add ice or sweeten with stevia to taste.

1. Process in a blender until smooth and serve immediately.

Option #4:
    1 cup fresh or frozen chopped strawberries
    1 frozen banana
    1-2 tablespoons ground flaxseeds or chia seeds
    1 scoop plant protein powder

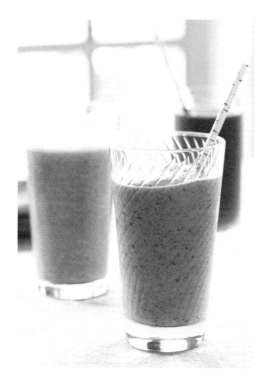

6 ounces coconut, almond, or skim milk
If desired, you may add ice or sweeten
with stevia to taste.

1. Process in a blender until smooth and serve immediately.

JUICY GRILLED CHICKEN BREASTS
Yield: 2 servings

You typically don't see the word "juicy" when describing a grilled boneless, skinless chicken breast, but in this case, it's deserved. The secret is pounding them thin, then allowing them to soak in an herbed brine solution before heading to the grill.

2 boneless, skinless chicken breasts
4 cups cold water
2 tablespoons sea or Himalayan salt
2 tablespoons sugar
2 sprigs fresh thyme
1 garlic clove, peeled and minced
1 tablespoon balsamic vinegar
1 tablespoon extra-virgin oil
Freshly cracked black pepper

6 ounces coconut, almond, or skim milk
If desired, you may add ice or sweeten
with stevia to taste.

1. Process in a blender until smooth and serve immediately.

Option #5:
1 cup frozen papayas, mangos, or
a combination
1-2 tablespoons ground flaxseeds or
chia seeds
1 scoop plant protein powder
1 tablespoon cashew nut or almond
butter

1. Place the chicken in a heavy-duty zip-top bag and seal.
2. With a meat mallet or rolling pin, pound the chicken to an even thickness of ¾ inch.
3. In a mixing bowl, whisk together the water, salt, sugar, and thyme.

4. Add the chicken breasts to mixture and refrigerate for 30 minutes.
5. Meanwhile, in a small bowl, whisk together the garlic, vinegar, and oil. Set aside.
6. Preheat the grill to medium-high.
7. Remove the chicken from the brine solution and discard the brine.
8. Pat the chicken dry and brush with the vinegar solution.
9. Grill for 5 minutes on each side or until browned.
10. Continue grilling until an instant read thermometer registers 160 degrees in the center.
11. Remove from the grill and let rest for at least 5 minutes.
12. Garnish with black pepper and serve warm.

Soothing Black Bean Soup
Yield: 6 servings

In order to enhance the look of this soup, the vegetables are cooked first. Canned black beans work just fine for this recipe, but it's even better if you use cooked dried beans.

1 tablespoon cumin seeds
2 tablespoons extra-virgin oil
2 large carrots, peeled and chopped
1 large sweet onion, peeled and chopped
1 large green bell pepper, seeded and chopped
1 large red bell pepper, seeded and chopped
1 large yellow bell pepper, seeded and chopped
3 garlic cloves, peeled and chopped
6 cups water
1 bay leaf
2 (15.5-ounce) cans black beans, drained and rinsed
2 tablespoons lemon juice
1 teaspoon seasoned salt
½ teaspoon ground coriander
½ teaspoon ground cumin
½ teaspoon black pepper
¼ teaspoon cayenne
Diced fresh tomato for garnish
Chopped fresh cilantro for garnish

1. Place the cumin seeds in a Dutch oven over medium-high heat.
2. Toast for 1 minute or until the seeds are fragrant.
3. Add the oil and when hot, stir in the carrots and chopped onion pieces.
4. Sauté for 2 minutes, stirring frequently.
5. Add the bell peppers and garlic.
6. Sauté 2 minutes longer.
7. Stir in the water, bay leaf, black beans, lemon juice, salt, coriander, ground cumin, black pepper, and cayenne.
8. Reduce the heat to low, cover, and cook for 35 minutes.
9. Remove from the heat and discard the bay leaf.
10. Serve warm with a garnish of diced tomato pieces and cilantro.

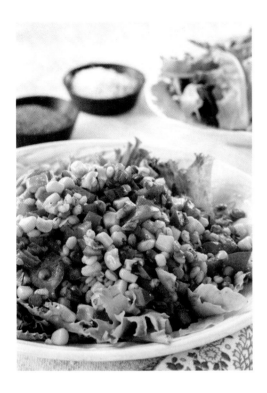

1 tablespoon balsamic vinegar

1 tablespoon extra-virgin oil

1 teaspoon lemon juice

½ teaspoon garlic salt

¼ teaspoon black pepper

Mixed salad greens

Crunchy Sweet Corn Salad
Yield: 2 servings

The summer sweetness of fresh corn with the crunch of pearl barley and lentils marries nicely in this seasonal salad. All three are cooked in the same pot. Serve it alone or over a bed of mixed greens.

¼ cup lentils

¼ cup pearl barley

2 ears sweet corn, shucked and silked

1 red bell pepper, seeded and chopped

1 green onion, chopped

1 tablespoon chopped fresh basil

1. Bring a large pot of water to a boil over high heat.
2. Stir in the barley and lentils and cook for 20 minutes.
3. Add the corn during the last 4 minutes of cooking.
4. Meanwhile, place the chopped bell pepper and onion pieces in a serving bowl.
5. In a separate bowl, whisk together the basil, vinegar, oil, juice, salt, and pepper. Set aside.
6. With tongs, remove the corn from the pot and set aside to cool slightly.
7. Drain the pot over a colander and rinse with cold water.
8. Drain thoroughly and add to the serving bowl.
9. Cut the kernels from the corn when cool enough to handle and add to the lentil mixture.
10. Whisk the dressing once more and add to the serving bowl.
11. Toss well to combine.
12. Set aside to meld at room temperature for 10 minutes before serving on a bed of mixed salad greens.

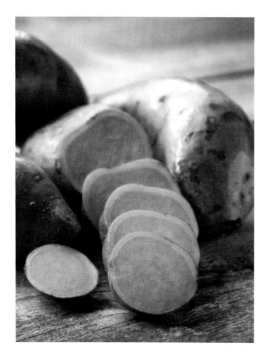

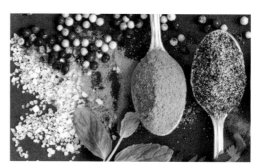

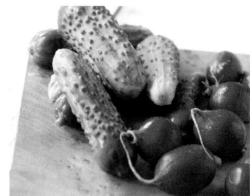

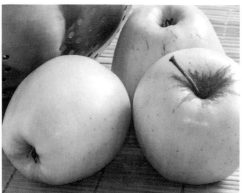

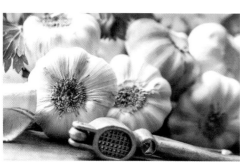

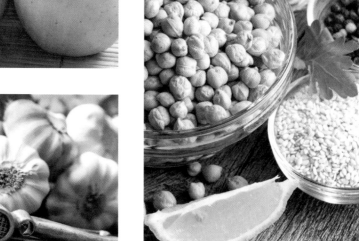

DAY 3

BREAK YOUR FAST HASH BROWNS
Yield: 2 servings

These look like traditional pan-fried hash browns, but they are actually baked in the oven. Get them going in the oven while you prepare for the day. You can substitute sweet potatoes for the regular potato if desired.

2 cups shredded baking potatoes
1 green onion, chopped
1 tablespoon cornstarch
⅛ teaspoon salt
⅛ teaspoon black pepper
⅛ teaspoon paprika

1. Place the potatoes in a bowl and cover with cold water. Let stand 5 minutes.
2. Meanwhile, preheat the oven to 475 degrees.
3. Line a baking sheet with parchment paper and grease with cooking spray. Set aside.
4. Drain the potatoes and pat dry with paper towels.
5. Dry the bowl and along with the potatoes, add the chopped onion pieces, cornstarch, salt, pepper, and paprika.
6. Place an open-ended round biscuit cutter on the prepared pan and fill with the potato mixture. Do not pack.
7. Carefully remove the cutter and repeat with the remaining mixture.
8. Lightly coat the tops with cooking spray.
9. Bake 20 minutes, turn and bake 12-15 minutes longer or until golden brown. Serve warm.

FOOD FACT: POTATOES

Storage: If you want to decrease the shelf life of a potato, wash it. That moisture will cause it to break down rapidly. Instead, place it in a cool, dark place. If it begins to sprout, simply pull off the shoots before preparing.

ROASTED NUT HUMMUS
Yield: 2 cups

As you know, roasting nuts changes the flavor beautifully. Adding those roasted nuts to a food processor along with hummus ingredients does the same thing for this spread or dip. You can use any nut variety you have on hand, but pecans or walnuts are magnificent!

1 (15.5-ounce) can chickpeas,
    drained and rinsed
1 garlic clove, peeled
½ cup coarsely chopped
    roasted nuts
3 tablespoons extra-virgin oil
3 tablespoons lemon juice
½ teaspoon ground cumin
¼ teaspoon lemon pepper
¼ teaspoon garlic salt
¼ teaspoon cayenne
⅛ teaspoon ground coriander

1. Place the chickpeas, garlic, nuts, oil, juice, cumin, lemon pepper, salt, cayenne, and coriander in the bowl of a food processor.
2. Process until smooth, stopping to scrape down the sides.
3. Transfer to a serving bowl or cover and refrigerate for later use.

Note: If you want a thinner hummus, add a tablespoon or two of water to the food processor.

ROOT SALAD
Yield: 3 servings

This recipe is deceiving because it looks like it took a long time to prepare but is actually very easy to make! Make the dressing ahead of time and it can literally be ready in minutes.

3 tablespoons white wine or apple cider
    vinegar
3 tablespoons nonfat Greek-style yogurt
2 tablespoons extra-virgin oil
½ teaspoon garlic or onion salt
¼ teaspoon black pepper
1 medium fennel bulb, trimmed and
    thinly sliced
1 small bunch watercress, trimmed
2 golden beets, peeled and coarsely
    grated
2 sunchokes or 1 jicama, peeled and
    thinly sliced
Mixed salad greens

1. In a small bowl, whisk together the vinegar, yogurt, oil, salt, and pepper. Set aside.
2. In a mixing bowl, gently stir together the fennel, beets, sunchokes, and watercress.
3. Drizzle with the dressing and serve over salad greens.

FOOD FACT: FENNEL

Selection: Even though I regularly see fennel as large as my hand, I gravitate to those that are small. In fact, I select the smallest I can find. They are easier to wash and you don't waste as much.

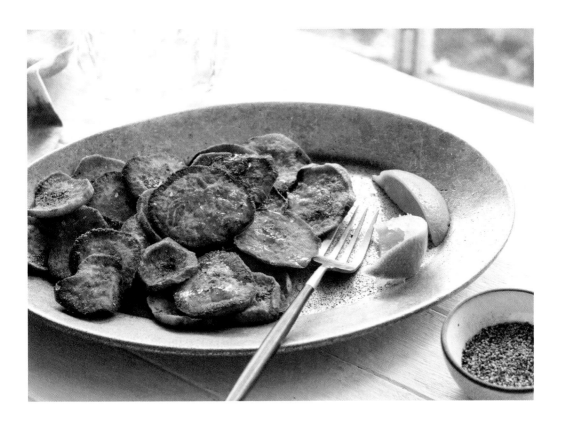

Sweet Potato "Fries" with Lime

Yield: 2 servings

Cilantro and fresh lime juice transform these oven fries into a side dish with pizazz. It is exceptional with grilled, baked, or broiled fish of any kind.

1 large sweet potato, cut in
    ¼-inch slices
1 tablespoon extra-virgin oil
¼ teaspoon garlic salt
¼ teaspoon coriander
⅛ teaspoon black pepper
⅛ teaspoon cayenne
½ lime

1. Preheat the oven to 375 degrees.
2. Lightly grease a baking sheet and add the sweet potato slices in a single layer.
3. In a small bowl, whisk together the oil, salt, coriander, pepper, and cayenne.
4. Drizzle mixture evenly over the sweet potato slices.
5. Bake 40–45 minutes or until tender and golden brown.
6. Immediately drizzle with the lime juice and serve warm.

CINNAMON BAKED APPLES
Yield: 2 servings

It is worth making this recipe for the aroma alone, but your taste buds will thank you with the first bite. It really can work double duty, as a side dish or dessert. You can have it baking away in the oven while you prepare dinner and have it as dessert.

    2 Golden Delicious apples
    ⅓ cup apple juice or water, divided
    2 teaspoons unsalted grass-fed butter,
        softened
    ½ teaspoon ground cinnamon
    ⅛ teaspoon ground nutmeg

1. Preheat the oven to 350 degrees.
2. Core the apples and place in a 9-inch pie plate.
3. In a small bowl, stir together 2 teaspoons of the apple juice, along with the butter, cinnamon, and nutmeg.
4. Evenly stuff mixture into the core of each apple.

5. Pour the remaining apple juice into the baking dish.
6. Bake 35 to 40 minutes or until the apples are tender. Serve warm.

CUCUMBER & RADISH SALAD
Yield: 3 servings

You will be amazed at the flavor and crunchy texture of this beautiful salad. Bonus: is it is super simple to prepare!

    2 tablespoons rice wine or apple cider
        vinegar
    1 tablespoon extra-virgin oil
    ¼ teaspoon garlic salt
    ⅛ teaspoon black pepper
    8 medium radishes, trimmed
        and thinly sliced
    3 green onions, trimmed and thinly
        sliced
    2 small cucumbers, thinly sliced
    3 tablespoons crumbled Feta cheese
    3 tablespoons chopped pecans

1. In a small bowl, whisk together the vinegar, oil, salt, and pepper. Set aside.
2. In a mixing bowl, toss together the radishes, onions, cucumbers, cheese, and pecans.
3. Drizzle the mixture with the dressing.
4. Cover and refrigerate at least 1 hour.
5. Serve with or without salad greens.

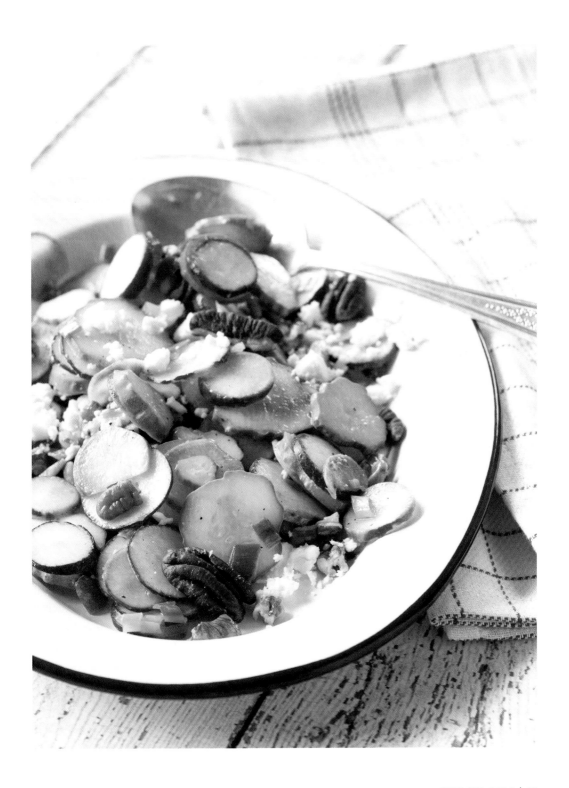

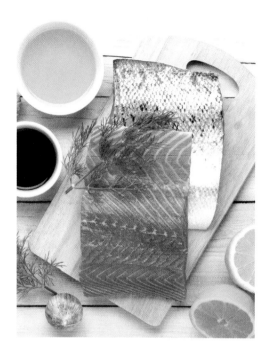

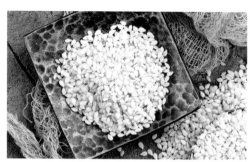

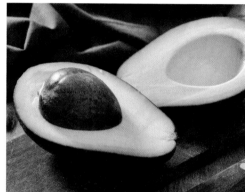

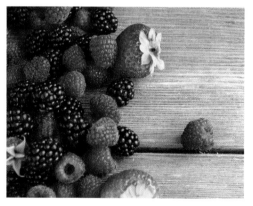

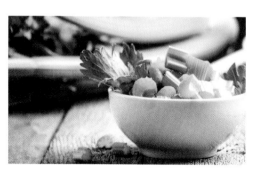

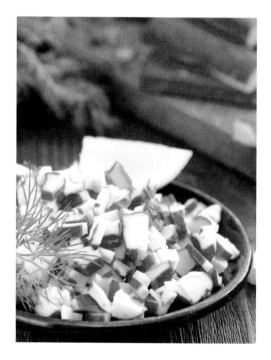

DAY 4

AVOCADO FRUIT SALAD WITH PINE NUTS
Yield: 2 servings

Salads that can transition with the seasons are a real treat! You can change this one depending on which fruits are in season. This is a salad that can take you from early spring all the way until fall.

    1 tablespoon extra-virgin oil
    2 tablespoons raspberry, white wine, or
        apple cider vinegar
    1 teaspoon honey
    ¼ teaspoon salt
    ⅛ teaspoon black pepper
    1 (8-ounce) package mixed salad
        greens
    1 ripe avocado, peeled, pitted, and
        cubed
    Juice of 1 lime
    1 cup coarsely chopped fruit
        (strawberries, raspberries, mangos,
        peaches, or papayas)
    2 tablespoons toasted pine nuts

1. In a small bowl, whisk together the oil, vinegar, honey, salt, and pepper. Set aside.
2. In a separate bowl, squeeze the lime juice over the avocado slices and set aside.
3. Divide the salad greens between two plates.
4. Top each with half of the chopped fruit and the avocado slices.
5. Drizzle evenly with the reserved dressing and garnish with the pine nuts.

FOOD FACT: STRAWBERRIES

Care: Do not wash or cap strawberries until you are ready to use. Think of strawberries as tiny sponges. Water will be absorbed by the fruit and break down the berry, so keep them unwashed in the refrigerator. Just before using, give them a gentle rinse with cold water. Drain in a colander or on paper towels then remove their green caps.

BARLEY VEGETABLE SOUP
Yield: 6 servings

It would be difficult to mess up this soup. It is aromatic, quick, and comes together in one pot. Plus, you can easily vary it with the produce you have on hand.

Substitutions: Dry herbs are more concentrated in flavor than fresh because all the moisture has been removed. To substitute fresh herbs for dried, use three times more than dried. There is one exception to this rule: Rosemary should be used in equal amounts. Use the formula in reverse when substituting dried for fresh herbs.

2 tablespoons extra-virgin oil
1 sweet onion, peeled and chopped
4 garlic cloves, peeled and minced
3 carrots, peeled and sliced
1 celery stalk, chopped
1 (8-ounce) package sliced mushrooms
8 cups low sodium vegetable or chicken stock (see page 96 or 117)
1 ¼ cups diced tomatoes
1 cup pearl barley
1 bay leaf
2 teaspoons dried thyme
1 teaspoon apple cider vinegar
½ teaspoon salt
¼ teaspoon black pepper
¼ teaspoon crushed red pepper

1. Place the oil in a Dutch oven over medium heat.
2. When hot, add the chopped onion pieces and garlic. Cook, stirring frequently for 3 minutes.
3. Add the carrots, celery, and mushrooms. Cook, stirring frequently for 6 minutes.
4. Add the stock, diced tomato pieces, barley, bay leaf, thyme, vinegar, salt, black pepper, and crushed red pepper.

5. Bring to a boil, then reduce the heat to low and simmer uncovered for 35 minutes or until the barley is tender.
6. Remove from the heat and discard the bay leaf. Serve warm.

SEARED TOFU WITH PEANUT DIPPING SAUCE
Yield: 2 servings

Searing tofu quickly allows the inside to remain nice and soft while the exterior is given a bit of body for easily handling. The dipping sauce is fairly addictive and is also great with carrot sticks.

¾ pound extra-firm tofu, drained
½ cup smooth natural peanut butter
¼ cup warm water
1-½ tablespoons red wine or apple cider vinegar
1 tablespoon lime juice
2 tablespoons extra-virgin oil, divided
1 garlic clove, peeled and minced
½ teaspoon crushed red pepper

1. Place the tofu between paper towels and gently press to remove any excess water.
2. Meanwhile, in a mixing bowl, vigorously whisk together the peanut butter and water until smooth.
3. Add the vinegar, lime juice, olive oil, garlic, and crushed red pepper to the mixing bowl. Set aside.
4. Place the tofu on a cutting board and cut into 4 slices.
5. Heat the remaining tablespoon olive oil in a skillet over high heat.
6. Add the tofu slices and sear until golden brown on one side, about 2 to 3 minutes.
7. Turn and brown the other side.
8. Serve warm with the peanut dipping sauce.

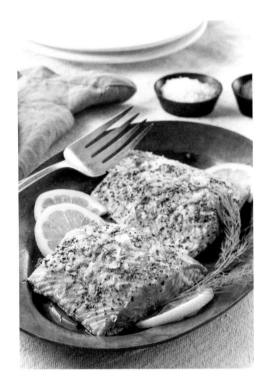

CITRUS HERB SALMON
Yield: 2 servings

This dish roasts in the oven and requires only one pan to clean. You can also wrap the fillets in parchment paper so they steam in their own juices. You can change the flavor completely by using lime juice instead of lemon and substituting chopped cilantro for the dill.

2 salmon fillets (around ½ pound total)
1 lemon
1 teaspoon chopped fresh dill (or fresh herb of your choice)
¼ teaspoon garlic salt
¼ teaspoon black pepper

1. Preheat the oven to 350 degrees.
2. Grease an 8x8-inch baking dish with cooking spray.
3. Add the fillets and spray the tops with cooking spray.
4. Cut the lemon in half and zest one half, then squeeze the juice from that half over the fillets.
5. Cut the remaining half into wedges for serving and set aside.
6. Sprinkle the fillets evenly with the zest, dill, salt, and pepper.
7. Roast for 20 minutes or until the salmon flakes easily with a fork.
8. Let rest 5 minutes before serving warm with the reserved lemon wedges.

Selection: Select sweet potatoes that are firm and have smooth, unblemished skins that are free of soft spots. Although they appear to be tough, they actually have thin skins that can tear easily, so handle with care.

SWEET POTATO MEDALLIONS
Yield: 2 servings

Nutrient rich sweet potatoes are simply peeled, sliced, and baked, but the end result tastes like there was much more effort. It only takes 30 minutes in the oven, so this makes it ideal for a weekend lunch or a weeknight dinner side dish. Leftovers are a great salad addition.

    1 large or 2 small sweet potatoes,
        peeled and cut in ½-inch slices
    1 tablespoon extra-virgin oil
    ⅛ teaspoon salt
    ⅛ teaspoon black pepper
    1 tablespoon chopped fresh parsley

1. Preheat the oven to 400 degrees.
2. Line a baking sheet with parchment paper and add the sweet potato slices in a single layer without touching.

3. Brush slices with the oil and sprinkle evenly with the salt and pepper.
4. Bake for 30 minutes or until just beginning to brown.
5. Remove from the oven and immediately sprinkle with the parsley. Serve warm.

BROILED CRAB CAKES
Yield: 3 servings

If you enjoy crabmeat, you probably appreciate a cake with less filling and more crab. That's exactly what you get here, as it bakes first, then browns under the oven broiler rather than being fried.

    ½ pound lump crab meat
    1 egg
    2 tablespoons whole wheat panko
    2 tablespoons chopped fresh parsley
    1-2 tablespoons diced pimentos,
        canned
    1 tablespoon plain non-fat yogurt
    2 teaspoon lime juice
    ¼ teaspoon black pepper
    ⅛ teaspoon cayenne or paprika

1. Preheat the oven to 425 degrees.
2. Cover a baking sheet with parchment and lightly grease with cooking spray.
3. In a mixing bowl, thoroughly combine the crab meat, egg white, panko, parsley, pimentos, yogurt, lime juice, pepper, and cayenne.

4. Form the mixture into 6 crab cakes and place 2 inches apart on the prepared baking sheet.
5. Slightly flatten and bake 10 minutes.
6. Remove from the oven and preheat the broiler to high.
7. Turn each cake over and broil until golden brown about 2 minutes.
Serve warm.

Option #2:
Mix the crab meat with:
2 tablespoons of light olive or avocado
    oil mayonnaise
½ teaspoon lemon pepper
¼ teaspoon cayenne
A pinch of salt and some chopped
    fresh dill
Prepare as directed above.

FOOD FACTS: CITRUS

Juicing: Always zest before squeezing! In order to get the most juice from any citrus product, make sure it is at room temperature. Then roll it back and forth on the counter while applying gentle pressure with your hand. It simply loosens up the fruit to allow more juice extraction.

Zesting: Don't go too crazy when zesting citrus. Just grate the outer colored peel of the fruit. Once you reach the white underneath, you'll get a bitter flavor rather than a citrus zing.

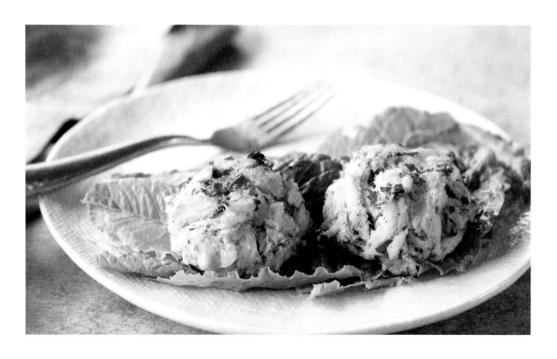

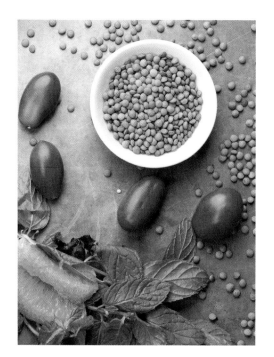
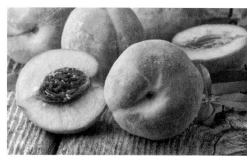
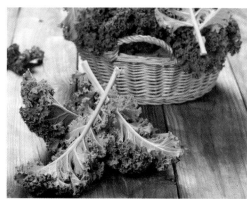
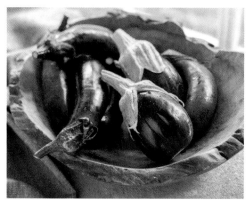
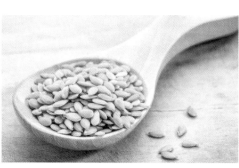
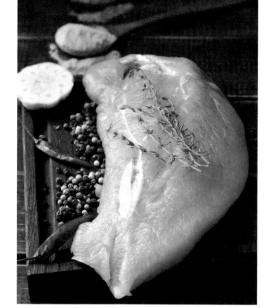

DAY 5

Tomato Lentil Salad
Yield: 4 servings

Enjoy this as a side salad or over salad greens. This is one of those salad mixtures that improves with age, so it will be even better the next day. The lemon and tarragon make it taste so fresh.

1 ¼ cups lentils
1 cup quartered cherry tomatoes
2 green onions, sliced
1 small yellow bell pepper, seeded
    and chopped
¼ cup extra-virgin oil
2 tablespoons lemon juice
2 garlic cloves, peeled and minced
1 tablespoon chopped fresh tarragon
1 teaspoon white wine or apple cider
    vinegar
1 teaspoon Dijon mustard
½ teaspoon lemon zest
½ teaspoon salt
¼ teaspoon black pepper
Mixed salad greens, optional

1. Bring a large pot of water to a boil over high heat.
2. Add the lentils, stir, and return to a boil.
3. Reduce the heat to low and simmer uncovered for 25 minutes or until the lentils are tender, but firm.
4. Drain lentils, shaking the colander to remove any excess moisture. Set pot aside to cool.
5. In a mixing bowl, combine the tomatoes, green onions, and chopped bell pepper pieces.
6. In a jar with a tight-fitting lid, combine the oil, lemon juice, garlic, tarragon, vinegar, mustard, zest, salt, and pepper.
7. Cover and shake well to emulsify.
8. Pour dressing over the tomato mixture and toss to evenly coat.
9. Add the lentils and mix well.
10. Chill or serve at room temperature.

FOOD FACTS: PEPPERS

Selection: Peppers should feel hard and crisp with a color that is glossy and quite vivid.

Storage: Peppers keep quite nicely in the refrigerator, but you'll know immediately when they begin to move past their prime. They fade and soften and start to wrinkle as they age.

Spaghetti Squash with Fresh Tomatoes & Kale
Yield: 2 servings

This dish may look like traditional spaghetti, but it is actually more nutritional. And, it tastes even better! The kale is wilted and spinach can be substituted, if desired.

 1 small spaghetti squash
 2 tomatoes, chopped
 1 tablespoon balsamic vinegar
 ½ teaspoon garlic salt
 ¼ teaspoon black pepper
 1 cup chopped fresh kale
 2 tablespoons crumbled Feta cheese

1. Cut the squash in half lengthwise.
2. Remove and discard the seeds and membranes.
3. Place the squash cut sides down in a Dutch oven and add water to a depth of 2 inches.
4. Place Dutch oven over medium-high heat and bring to a boil.
5. Cover, reduce the heat to low, and simmer 20 minutes or until the squash is easily pierced with a knife.
6. Meanwhile, place the tomatoes in a small bowl and drizzle with the vinegar. Toss well and sprinkle with the salt and pepper and set aside.
7. Place the kale in a serving bowl.
8. Drain Dutch oven and let cool for 5 minutes.
9. With a fork, remove the spaghetti-like strands and place onto the kale.
10. Discard the outer squash shell and allow the strands to wilt the kale.
11. Add the tomatoes and juices, tossing well.
12. Sprinkle with the Feta and serve warm.

FOOD FACT: SQUASH (WINTER)

Storage: These vegetables have an incredibly long shelf life and do quite well at room temperature. I like to consume them within a few weeks.

Fresh Fruit Granita
Yield: 2 servings

This frozen dessert is made for the dog days of summer, and you can use practically any fruit you have on hand. Cantaloupe, honeydew, watermelon, and peaches are fantastic! Whipping as the mixture freezes breaks up the ice crystals and gives it a shaved ice texture.

 5 cups cubed fruit
 3 to 4 tablespoons lime juice
 1 tablespoon water
 Fresh mint for garnish

1. Place the fruit, juice, and water in the bowl of a food processor and puree until smooth.
2. Transfer puree to a shallow container, cover, and place in the freezer for one hour.
3. After 1 hour, whisk puree to break up any ice crystals.
4. Repeat freezing and whisking 3 times every 45 minutes.
5. Serve in chilled glasses with a garnish of fresh mint.

SAVORY HERB MUFFINS
Yield: about 12 muffins

This recipe is quick and easy. These muffins can be on the table from start to finish in 30 minutes. Place them in the oven while preparing the rest of the meal so they will be a warm addition. Use your favorite herb or a mixture, like chives, tarragon, and parsley.

2 cups gluten-free all-purpose flour
¼ cup chopped fresh herbs
1 tablespoon baking powder
½ teaspoon salt
¼ teaspoon black pepper
1¼ cups almond, coconut, or nonfat milk
⅓ cup extra-virgin oil
1 tablespoon Dijon mustard

1. Preheat the oven to 375 degrees.
2. Line 12 muffin cups with paper liners and set aside.

3. In a mixing bowl, stir together the flour, herbs, baking powder, salt, and pepper.
4. In a separate bowl, whisk together the milk, oil, and mustard.
5. Make a well in the center of the dry ingredients and add the milk mixture.
6. Stir just until blended.
7. Evenly divide the batter among the muffin cups, filling no more than two-thirds full.
8. Bake 18-21 minutes or until a cake tester inserted in the center comes out clean. The tops will be golden brown.
9. Let cool 2 minutes, then transfer to a wire rack to cool completely or enjoy while still warm.

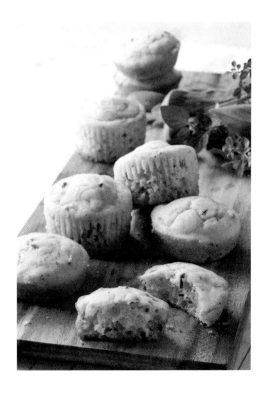

GRILLED VEGETABLE SOUP
Yield: 6 servings

Taking summer vegetables back outside and placing them on the grill completely changes their flavor. In this case, it's red bell peppers, onions, and eggplant. The eggplant in particular gives this soup a hearty, filling texture that freezes exceptionally well.

   2 large eggplant, peeled and cut in
       1-inch thick slices
   2 large red bell peppers
   2 large sweet onions, peeled and
       quartered
   2½ tablespoons extra-virgin oil, divided
   6 large garlic cloves, peeled and
       minced
   2 celery stalks, chopped
   2 carrots, peeled and chopped
   6 cups vegetable stock (preferably
       homemade [see page 96], but low
       sodium if purchased)

   2 large tomatoes, peeled and
       chopped
   2 tablespoons chopped fresh basil
   2 teaspoons fresh thyme
   ½ teaspoon onion or garlic salt
   ¼ teaspoon paprika
   ¼ teaspoon black pepper

1. Preheat the grill to medium heat.
2. Brush the eggplant, peppers, and onions with 1-½ tablespoons of the oil.
3. Place the eggplant and onions in a grill pan or skewer the onions, if desired.
4. Place on the rack and grill for 4 to 5 minutes, turning halfway through. You want the eggplant and onions to have nice grill marks and the peppers to be blistered.
5. Place the eggplant and onions in a baking dish and set aside.
6. Place the peppers in a deep bowl and cover with plastic wrap to steam.
7. When the eggplant and onions are cool enough to handle, coarsely chop and set aside along with any accumulated juices. Set for 5 minutes.
8. After 5 minutes, remove the plastic wrap from the pepper container. Peel away and discard the dark outer skin, seeds and pith.
9. Coarsely chop the peppers.
10. Place the remaining oil in a Dutch oven over medium-high heat.
11. When hot, add the garlic, celery, and carrots.

12. Sauté for 5 minutes, stirring frequently.
13. Add the stock, tomatoes, and the grilled vegetables, along with any liquid created.
14. Cook for 10 minutes and add the basil, thyme, salt, paprika, and pepper.
15. Cook 2 minutes longer and serve warm.

TURKEY & FLAXSEED MEATBALLS
Yield: 14 meatballs

You'll never cook meatballs the same after tasting this recipe! You can also make these meatballs with ground chicken, but will likely return to turkey, it's that good. And, conveniently, whole wheat breadcrumbs are now widely available at most supermarkets. Instead of serving these with marinara sauce, place them on a thick slice of tomato. Bonus: leftovers freeze beautifully.

   1 pound extra lean ground turkey
   2 garlic cloves, peeled and minced
   1 (10-ounce) package frozen spinach, thawed and squeezed dry
   1 egg, beaten
   ¾ cup panko, whole wheat, or gluten-free breadcrumbs
   ¼ cup crumbled Feta cheese
   2 tablespoons ground flaxseeds
   1 teaspoon dried oregano
   ¼ teaspoon black pepper
   1 tomato, thickly sliced

1. Preheat the oven to 375 degrees.
2. Place a wire rack on a large baking sheet and coat lightly with cooking spray. Set aside.
3. In a mixing bowl, combine the turkey, garlic, spinach, egg, breadcrumbs, cheese, flaxseeds, oregano, and pepper.
4. With your hands, form into 14 meatballs and place on the prepared rack.
5. Bake 30 minutes or until the meatballs have reached an internal temperature of 165 degrees.
6. Remove from the oven and let stand 10 minutes before serving on top of tomato slices.

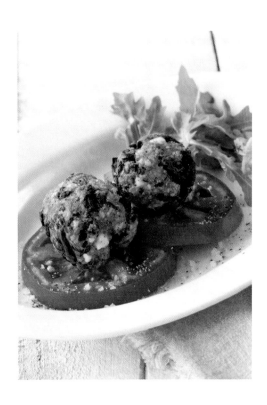

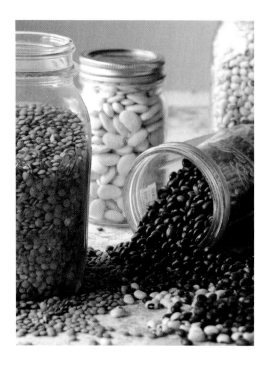

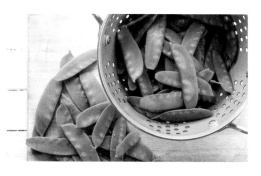

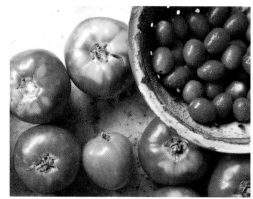

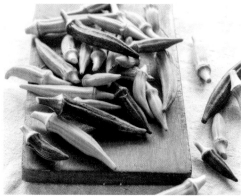

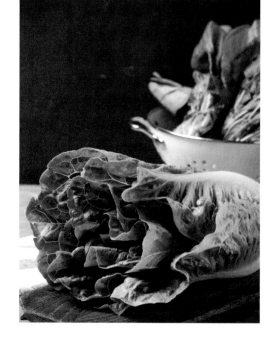

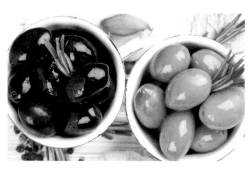

DAY 6

DRY BEAN/PEA COOKING PRIMER
Yield: 6 to 8 servings

Bags of dry beans are possibly the most inexpensive item you can purchase at the supermarket. For pennies, you can rehydrate them to use in soups, as a side dish, and on top of salads. Use this guide for any dry bean varieties. The exception? Lentils and split peas that don't require soaking.

    1 (1-pound) package dry beans or peas

Traditional Soak:
1. Pour the dry beans or peas in a large bowl and cover with 6 cups of cold water.
2. Let stand at room temperature for 8 hours or overnight.
3. Drain, rinse, and cook the beans or peas with fresh water.

Quick Soak:
1. Pour the dry beans or peas in a large saucepan and cover with cold water by 2 inches.
2. Place over high heat and bring to a boil.
3. Boil for 2 minutes, remove from the heat, cover and let stand for 1 hour.
4. Drain, rinse, and cook the beans or peas with fresh water.

FOOD FACT: GARLIC

Selection: Garlic bulbs should have papery outer skins and never have any evidence of sprouting. If they are soft, they are old and should be discarded and certainly not purchased.

SPICED LENTIL DIP
Yield: 2 ¼ cups

If possible, when at the grocery store, search for either red or yellow lentils for this dip, and you'll love the look. It is spicy but not so much that it will send you running for the water faucet. Use it with any raw veggies, and in the summer months, garnish it with chopped grape tomatoes.

    2 teaspoons extra-virgin oil
    1 large shallot, peeled and chopped
    4 garlic cloves, peeled and minced
    1 teaspoon curry powder
    ½ teaspoon ground cumin
    ½ teaspoon salt
    ¼ teaspoon ground coriander
    ¼ teaspoon crushed red pepper
    ⅛ teaspoon black pepper

2 cups cooked lentils, room temperature
2 tablespoons lemon juice
Chopped fresh parsley for garnish

1. Place the oil in a small skillet over medium-high heat.
2. When hot, add the chopped shallot pieces and garlic.
3. Cook 2 minutes, stirring frequently.
4. Add the curry powder, cumin, salt, coriander, crushed red pepper, and black pepper. Cook 2 minutes longer or until fragrant.
5. Meanwhile, place the lentils and lemon juice in a food processor.
6. Add the skillet mixture and process until smooth.
7. Transfer to a serving bowl and allow to cool to room temperature or cover and refrigerate until ready to serve.

HOMEMADE LOW SODIUM VEGETABLE STOCK
Yield: 8 cups

With this easy recipe, there is no reason not to make your own stock to use in soups and stews. Making it in a slow cooker allows the mixture to simmer away while you are doing other things. It only demands that you strain it at the end of the day. As you cook other recipes, simply save the tops, ends and peelings from celery, carrots, parsnips, onions (not the papery portion), bell peppers, shallots, green onions, and leeks, as well as the stems of fresh herbs. You can collect the scraps in a large zip-top bag that stays in the freezer. Then when you have enough, it is transformed into the basis for delicious meals.

5 cups frozen vegetable scraps
8 cups water
2 bay leaves
1 teaspoon black peppercorns
½ teaspoon salt

1. Place the vegetable scraps in a large slow cooker.
2. Add the water, bay leaves, peppercorns, and salt.
3. Cover and cook on low for 8 hours or on high for 4 hours.
4. Cool completely and strain with a fine mesh sieve.
5. Discard solids.
6. Refrigerate and use within 4 days or package into freezer containers and freeze.

FOOD FACTS: PARSNIPS

Season: Once frost has hit the plant, you'll have a sweeter root since the starch turns to sugar.

Selection: I like small parsnips because overly large roots tend to have a woody center. They should feel firm like carrots.

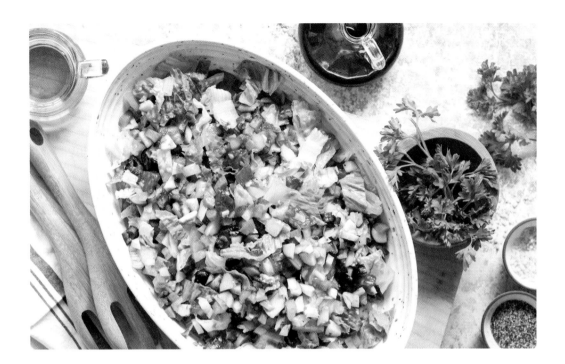

Lunch Time Chopped Salad
Yield: 2 servings

This is a great "clean out the crisper drawer" salad that can use up all those accumulated odds and ends of vegetables. Because everything is chopped and mixed together, it's super portable for a lunch on the go or at your desk.

2 hearts of romaine, coarsely chopped

1 cucumber, chopped

1 large tomato, diced

1 shallot, peeled and chopped

1 small carrot, peeled and finely
  chopped

1 yellow bell pepper, seeded and
  chopped

4 pitted black olives, chopped

2 tablespoons chopped fresh parsley

2 tablespoons extra-virgin oil

1 tablespoon balsamic vinegar

½ teaspoon salt

¼ teaspoon black pepper

Roasted okra slices for garnish

1. Place the hearts of romaine, diced tomato, chopped cucumber, shallot, carrot, and pepper pieces, olives, and parsley in a mixing bowl.
2. Drizzle with the oil and vinegar.
3. Sprinkle with the salt and pepper.
4. Toss to evenly coat.
5. Cover and refrigerate for later use or serve immediately with a garnish of roasted okra slices.

FOOD FACTS: CUCUMBERS

Selection: Buy cucumbers when they are firm and as solid bright green as possible.

Storage: Cucumbers will exist happily in a loosely closed plastic bag in the refrigerator for a week or longer.

ICED CUCUMBER SOUP
Yield: 4 servings

Starting in the early summer, cucumbers hit the market quickly and frequently, which means they are economical for quite some time. Local supplies come to a halt at the first frost. This chilled soup helps keep you cool during the hottest weeks of the year.

    3 large cucumbers, peeled and seeded
    1 cup plain non-fat yogurt
    1 garlic clove, peeled
    1½ tablespoons extra-virgin oil
    2 teaspoons white wine, apple cider,
        or champagne vinegar
    1 tablespoon chopped fresh mint
    1 teaspoon salt
    ¼ teaspoon black pepper
    Greek yogurt for garnish
    Mint sprigs for garnish

1. Place the cucumbers, yogurt, garlic, oil, vinegar, mint, salt, and pepper in a blender or food processor.
2. Blend until smooth and transfer to a serving bowl.
3. Cover and refrigerate for at least 1 hour.
4. Serve cold with a dollop of yogurt and mint sprigs.

EARLY SUMMER VEGETABLES WITH ROASTED ALMONDS
Yield: 2 servings

Think green when you visualize this side dish because it combines every shade in this delicious vegetable stir fry. You will love it with roasted chicken or turkey.

    1½ cups snow peas
    1 tablespoon extra-virgin oil
    1 large leek, sliced
    1 small cucumber, peeled and cut in
        ½-inch strips
    1 lime, zested and juiced
    ¼ teaspoon white pepper
    ¼ cup sliced, roasted almonds
    Chopped fresh parsley for garnish

1. Place the snow peas in a saucepan and cover with hot water.
2. Place over high heat and bring to a boil.
3. Cook for 1 minute or until the peas are vibrant green and slightly puffed.
4. Drain well and set aside.

5. Place the oil in a large skillet over medium-high heat.
6. When hot, add the leeks and cook 3 minutes, stirring frequently.
7. Stir in the cucumber strips and lime zest and cook another 5 minutes.
8. Stir in the reserved snow peas, lime juice, pepper, and almonds.
9. Cook 1 minute longer and serve warm with a garnish of fresh parsley.

FOOD FACTS: LEEKS

Washing: Clean leeks by cutting off the coarser green leaves. Split the leek down the middle so that any grit can be quickly washed away. Then trim and chop or slice as desired.

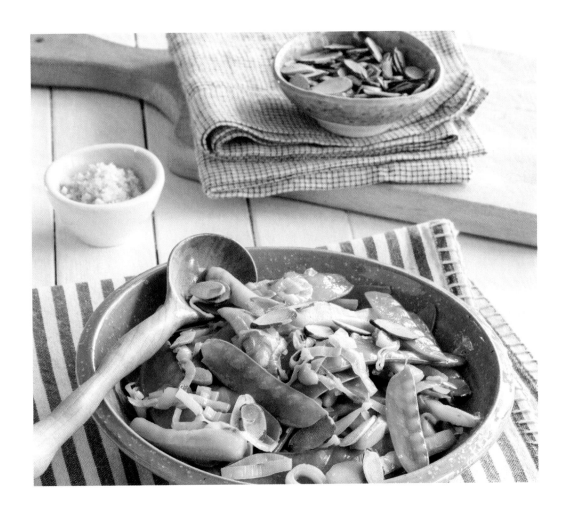

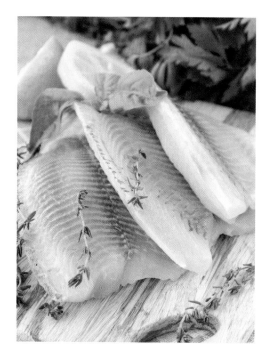
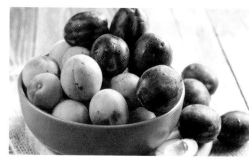
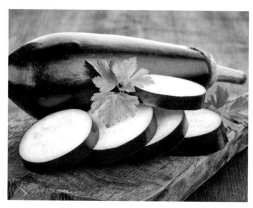
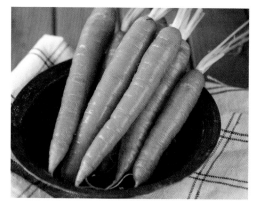
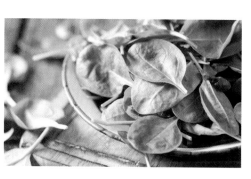
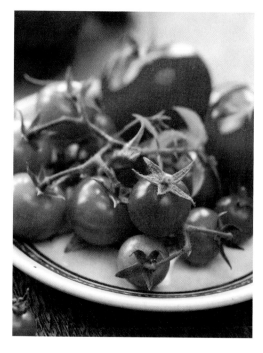

DAY 7

OVEN-ROASTED SUMMER FRUIT
Yield: 2 servings

Peaches, nectarines, apricots, plums, figs, oh my! And all can be beautifully roasted in the oven. What does roasting do? It naturally caramelizes while softening the fruit. It's fantastic alone or served with a dollop of Greek yogurt.

- 1 tablespoon unsalted, grass-fed butter
- 1-2 teaspoon stevia
- ¼ teaspoon pure vanilla or almond extract
- 2 peaches, nectarines, or apricots, halved and pitted or 4 ripe plums or figs, halved

1. Place the butter in an 8x8-inch baking dish and place in the oven.
2. Preheat the oven to 425 degrees, watching to remove the baking dish as soon as the butter completely melts.
3. Allow the oven to finish preheating.
4. Sprinkle the stevia over the melted butter and add the extract. Stir until the stevia dissolves.
5. Place the fruit cut side down in the baking dish.
6. Roast for 8 minutes, then turn over and roast another 4 minutes. Serve warm.

FOOD FACT: PLUMS

Pitting: Some plum varieties are freestone (just like peaches) and the pits pop out easily. Others are semi-cling and clingstone. Treat them just as you would fresh peaches and cut around the pit for slices if it doesn't remove promptly.

LIGHT COLESLAW
Yield: 2 servings

This deliciously crisp coleslaw goes with everything from poultry to fish. It really stands out thanks to dividing the addition of the cabbage, with some stirred into the mixture just as it is being served.

- 1 tablespoon celery seeds
- 3 cups shredded cabbage
- 1 carrot, peeled and grated
- ½ cup apple cider vinegar
- 2 tablespoons light mayonnaise
- ¼ teaspoon salt
- ¼ teaspoon white pepper

1. Place the celery seeds in a small dry skillet over medium heat.

2. Dry roast for 2 minutes or until fragrant and set aside to cool.
3. Meanwhile, in a mixing bowl, combine 2½ cups of the cabbage and the grated carrot.
4. In a separate bowl, whisk together the vinegar, mayonnaise, salt, and pepper.
5. Add the cooled celery seeds and add to the cabbage mixture.
6. Toss to evenly coat, cover, and refrigerate at least 30 minutes.
7. When ready to serve, stir in the remaining cabbage.

FOOD FACT: CARROTS

Selection: I prefer to purchase carrots in bundles with their feathery tops attached over those packaged in plastic bags. It allows me to feel them for firmness, and I can tell by the tops how fresh they are.

SPINACH & LENTIL SOUP
Yield: 6 servings

This soup can be practically instant if you chop the vegetables ahead of time. Quick-cooking lentils allow this soup to be ready in less than 30 minutes.

1 tablespoon extra-virgin oil
4 celery stalks, chopped
1 large sweet onion, peeled and chopped
3 garlic cloves, peeled and minced
3 carrots, peeled and chopped
6 cups low sodium, organic vegetable or chicken stock (see page 96 or 117)
2 cups lentils
1 bay leaf
1 teaspoon dried basil
1 teaspoon seasoned salt
½ teaspoon dried thyme
½ teaspoon dried chives
¼ teaspoon black pepper
¼ teaspoon paprika
4 cups baby spinach leaves, coarsely chopped
Chopped fresh parsley for garnish

1. Place the oil in a Dutch oven over medium-high heat.
2. When hot, add the chopped onion pieces, garlic, celery, and carrots.
3. Sauté 3 minutes or until the vegetables soften.
4. Add the stock, lentils, bay leaf, basil, salt, thyme, chives, pepper, and paprika.
5. Bring to a boil, then reduce the heat to low, cover, and simmer for 20 minutes.
6. If necessary, add 1 cup of hot water along with the baby spinach.
7. Cook 2 minutes longer to allow the spinach to wilt.
8. Remove from the heat and discard the bay leaf.
9. Serve warm with a garnish of fresh parsley.

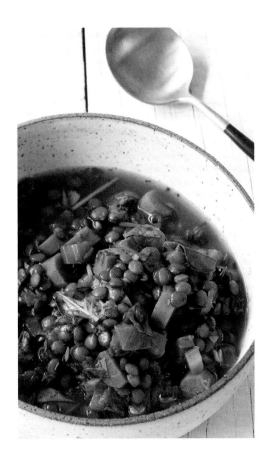

PLANK GRILLED FISH WITH FRESH HERB RUB
Yield: 2 servings

It takes a bit of forethought to pull off this recipe only because you need to soak the wood planks in water for an hour before grilling. Consider using alder, hickory, or cedar. Then utilize any whitefish you desire, such as haddock or flounder. The fresh herb rub is also terrific on grilled turkey, chicken, or pork.

2 wood planks
2 whitefish fillets
¼ teaspoon seasoned salt
¼ teaspoon paprika
¼ teaspoon black pepper
1 teaspoon chopped fresh thyme
1 teaspoon chopped fresh parsley
½ teaspoon chopped fresh chives
Juice of ½ lime

1. Soak wood planks in water for one hour.
2. Preheat the grill to medium-high.
3. Remove the planks from the soaking water and lightly spray both sides with cooking spray.
4. Place the fillets on a baking sheet.
5. In a small bowl, combine the salt, paprika, and pepper.
6. Sprinkle evenly over both sides of the fish, rubbing it into the fillets.
7. In a small bowl, combine the thyme, parsley, chives, and lime juice. Set aside.
8. Place the planks on the grill grate and allow to heat on one side for 3 minutes.
9. Flip the planks over and place the fillets on top.
10. Cover and grill for 12 minutes or until the fish is opaque and flakes easily with a fork.
11. Remove fish from the planks and transfer to a serving plate.
12. Remove planks from grill.
13. Smear fish on one side with the herb rub and serve immediately.

ARUGULA WITH GRILLED OKRA & TOMATOES
Yield: 2 servings

If you've ever had a vegetable garden, you know that harvesting cherry tomatoes and okra can be a daily job for the hottest couple of months. Since both vegetables like the summer heat, place them on the grill while you have it fired up for other things. The char will enhance a simple salad and go with anything else you have on the menu. A grilling basket really helps with this recipe.

    1 pint cherry tomatoes
    1 pound small okra
    3 tablespoons extra-virgin oil, divided
    ½ teaspoon seasoned salt
    ¼ teaspoon black pepper
    Arugula
    2 tablespoons balsamic vinegar

1. Preheat the grill to medium-high.
2. Meanwhile, place the tomatoes and okra in a mixing bowl.
3. Drizzle with 1 tablespoon of oil and the salt and pepper.
4. Toss well to evenly coat and transfer to a grilling basket.
5. Scatter the vegetables so they are in a single layer. Grill for 3 minutes with the grill covered.
6. Place the arugula in a serving bowl and add the grilled vegetables.
7. Toss well with the remaining oil and vinegar. Serve immediately.

CAPONATA
Yield: 3 ½ cups

This is a versatile recipe! Eggplant is the basis for this snack that can also be a wrap ingredient or served over mixed salad greens. Serve it with toasted gluten-free pita bread or baked tortilla chips (see page 125). This is a make-ahead dish, and leftovers can be easily frozen for later use.

    1 tablespoon extra-virgin oil
    1 pound eggplant, peeled and diced
    4 green onions, trimmed and sliced

3 celery stalks, chopped

1 red bell pepper, minced

2 large garlic cloves, peeled and minced

1 (8-ounce) can low sodium tomato sauce (or homemade)

¼ cup chopped black olives

3 tablespoons low sodium tomato paste

2 tablespoons red wine or apple cider vinegar

1 tablespoon stevia

¼ teaspoon dried oregano

¼ teaspoon black pepper

1. Place the oil in a large saucepan over medium heat.
2. When hot, add the eggplant, onions, celery, bell peppers, and garlic.
3. Cook 10 minutes, stirring frequently.
4. Stir in the tomato sauce, olives, tomato paste, vinegar, stevia, oregano, and pepper.
5. Cook 20 minutes, remove from the heat, and allow to cool to room temperature.
6. Cover and chill for 8 hours. Bring to room temperature when ready to serve.

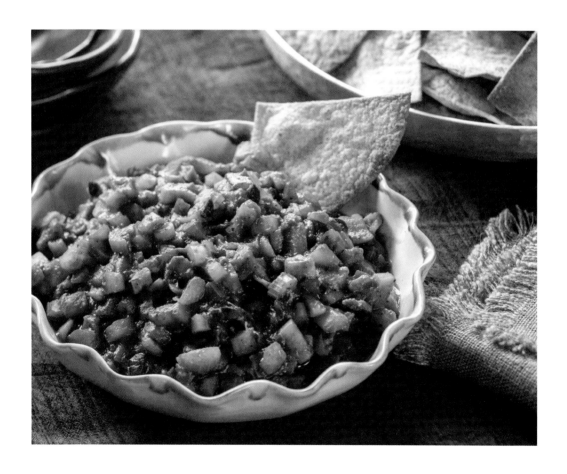

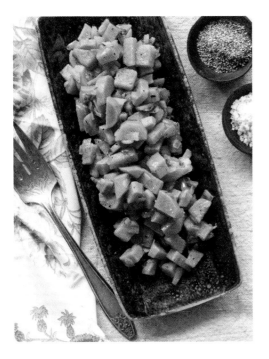

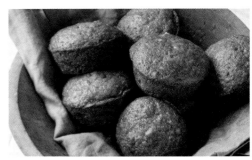

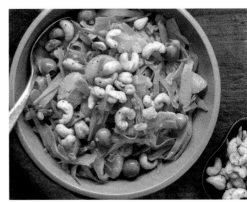

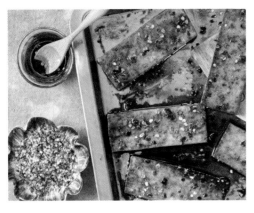

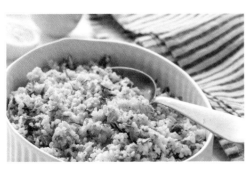

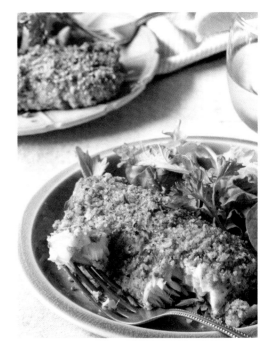

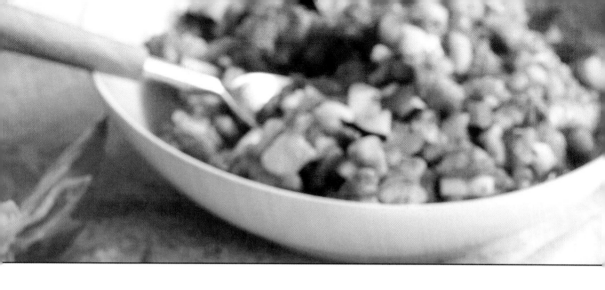

WEEK TWO

Days 8–14

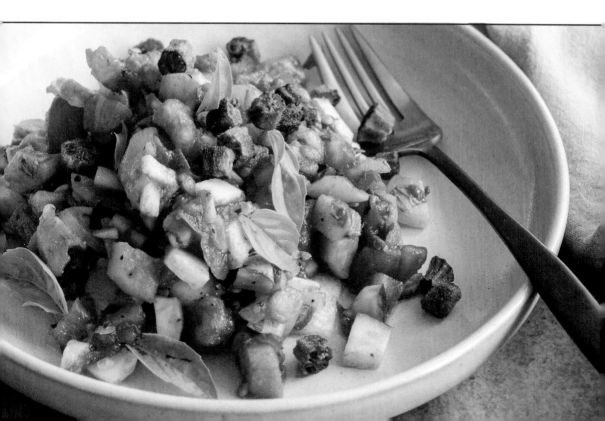

SHOPPING LIST – WEEK 2

(DAYS 8–14)

FRUIT

- [ ] Bananas – 4
- [ ] Blackberries – 6-ounce package
- [ ] Blueberries – 6-ounce package
- [ ] Fig – 1
- [ ] Grapefruit – 1
- [ ] Mango – 1
- [ ] Nectarine or Peach – 1
- [ ] Pineapple – 1 small
- [ ] Plum or Tangerine – 1
- [ ] Strawberries – 16-ounce package

VEGETABLES

- [ ] Avocados – 2
- [ ] Broccoli – 7 day supply
- [ ] Brussels Sprouts – 1 serving size
- [ ] Cucumbers – 7 day supply
- [ ] Eggplant – 2
- [ ] English Peas – 1 serving size
- [ ] Fennel – 1 bulb
- [ ] Green Beans – 7 day supply
- [ ] Mushrooms – 7 day supply
- [ ] Okra – 1 serving size
- [ ] Peppers (variety of colors) – 7 day supply
- [ ] Salad Greens (chicory, spinach, kale, Belgian endive, bean sprouts, iceberg, romaine) – 7 day supply for twice daily salads
- [ ] Spinach – 7 day supply
- [ ] Sugar Snap Peas – 1 serving size
- [ ] Swiss Chard – 1 serving size bunch
- [ ] Tomatoes – 7 day supply

CANNED & PACKAGED

- [ ] Hummus – 6-ounce container

MEAT

- [ ] Boneless, Skinless Chicken Breast – 5*
- [ ] Extra Lean Beef (96/4, petite fillet) – 2*
- [ ] Catfish Fillet*
- [ ] Crawfish*
- [ ] Shrimp (large)*
- [ ] Salmon Fillet*
- [ ] Scallops*
- [ ] Tilapia Fillet*
- [ ] Turkey Breast Tenderloin*

amount varies by gender
(see meal plan)

PESTICIDES IN FRUITS AND VEGETABLES

The amount of pesticides in fruits and vegetables depends on several factors, including the type of plant, how it grows, its skin, how it's watered, and the length of the growing season. According to the Environmental Working Group (EWP), there is a "Dirty Dozen" of fruits/vegetables with higher amounts of pesticides and a "Clean Fifteen" of fruits/vegetables with lower amounts of pesticides.

The Dirty Dozen:	The Clean Fifteen:
1. Apples	1. Avocados
2. Peaches	2. Sweet corn
3. Nectarines	3. Pineapples
4. Strawberries	4. Cabbage
5. Grapes	5. Sweet peas (frozen)
6. Celery	6. Onions
7. Spinach	7. Asparagus
8. Sweet bell peppers	8. Mangos
9. Cucumbers	9. Papayas
10. Cherry tomatoes	10. Kiwi
11. Snap peas (imported)	11. Eggplant
12. Potatoes	12. Grapefruit
	13. Cantaloupe
	14. Cauliflower
	15. Sweet potatoes

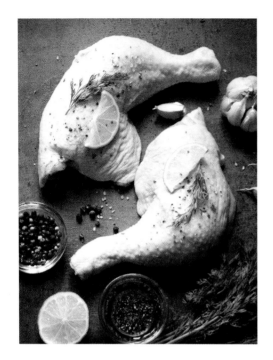

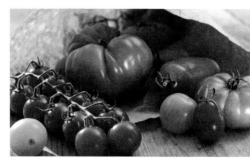

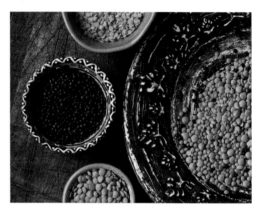

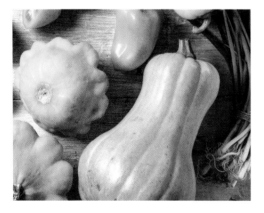

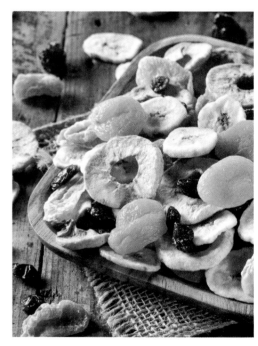

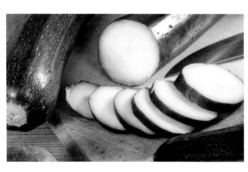

DAY 8

Beef & Barley Soup
Yield: 6 servings

This is one of the most nourishing soups you can make, and luckily this recipe makes a lot. You will never tire of it, no matter how many times it is reheated, and you can freeze the excess.

1 pound lean ground chuck

1 quart water

1 (15-ounce) can stewed tomatoes (select low or no salt added)

1 (6-ounce) can low sodium tomato juice cocktail

1 small sweet onion, peeled and chopped

1 large carrot, peeled and chopped

3 celery stalks, chopped

2 large garlic cloves, peeled and minced

1 cup low sodium vegetable or beef stock

⅓ cup dried barley

⅓ cup dried split peas

1 bay leaf

¼ teaspoon black pepper

¼ teaspoon dried basil

¼ teaspoon dried oregano

¼ teaspoon paprika

1. In a large Dutch oven over medium-high heat, brown the chuck, breaking apart any large pieces as it cooks.
2. When thoroughly cooked, drain on paper towels and pat dry. Wipe away any pan drippings left in the pot with a paper towel.
3. Return the meat to the Dutch oven and add the water, tomatoes, juice, chopped onion and carrot pieces, celery, garlic, stock, barley, peas, bay leaf, pepper, basil, oregano, and paprika. Stir well and bring to a boil.
4. Cover and reduce the heat to low. Simmer for 1 hour.
5. Remove from the heat, discard the bay leaf, and serve warm.

FOOD FACT: ONIONS

Cutting: Always use a sharp knife when cutting onions of any type. A dull knife will destroy more of the onion's structure, causing it to release more of the sulfur-containing amino acids. It's these acids that not only make you cry when chopping, but give onions a stronger aroma.

ROASTED BANANAS
Yield: 2 servings

During the winter when all other fruits are either at a premium, tasteless, or non-existent, this is my go-to treat. With just a little heat, you can transform bananas. The key is to completely preheat the oven.

> 2 bananas
> 1 teaspoon unsalted, grass-fed butter, room temperature

1. Preheat the oven to 400 degrees.
2. Meanwhile, leaving the peel attached, slice the bananas in half lengthwise.
3. Place on an ungreased baking sheet with the cut side up.
4. Evenly smear each cut half with butter.
5. Bake 9-10 minutes or until the bananas are golden brown. Serve warm.

FOOD FACT: BANANAS

Not Ripe Enough: Soft, brown, or brown-speckled skins on a banana indicate sweetness and are perfect for baking. If your bananas are still too hard and you need them softer, just peel the fruit and place on an ungreased baking sheet. Oven bake them at 450 degrees for 10 minutes and then cool. They will be ready to mash and use.

EARLY FALL SQUASH & PEPPERS
Yield: 3 servings

This dish looks like sunshine on a rainy day. The butternut squash is roasted, then adorned with yellow bell pepper slices and a lemon honey dressing. It sings alongside roasted pork.

> 1 small butternut squash, peeled, seeded, and cut in ½-inch slices
> 2 garlic cloves, peeled and minced
> 1 tablespoon extra-virgin oil
> 6 fresh thyme sprigs
> 1 teaspoon extra-virgin oil
> 1 large yellow bell pepper, seeded and cut in ½-inch slices
> ¼ cup whole almonds
> 1 teaspoon stevia
> 1 lemon, zested and juiced
> ⅛ teaspoon white pepper

1. Preheat the oven to 400 degrees.
2. Place the squash on a lightly greased baking sheet in a single layer.
3. Sprinkle with the garlic and olive oil.
4. Top with the thyme sprigs and roast for 20 minutes.
5. Meanwhile, when the squash has about 10 minutes remaining, place the oil in a large skillet over medium-high heat.
6. When hot, add the bell pepper slices and cook for 5 minutes, stirring frequently.

7. Transfer pepper slices with a slotted spoon to a serving dish and add the almonds, stevia, lemon zest, lemon juice, and pepper to the skillet. Stir constantly until the stevia has melted.
8. Transfer the squash to the serving dish and drizzle with the glaze. Toss gently and serve warm.

DRIED FRUIT MUFFINS
Yield: about 16 muffins

This recipe works great with any type of dried fruit you have on hand, but using dried peaches or apricots is perfect.

Note: Change the zest to lime if using dried pineapple and to lemon if you use dried blueberries, cranberries, or cherries.

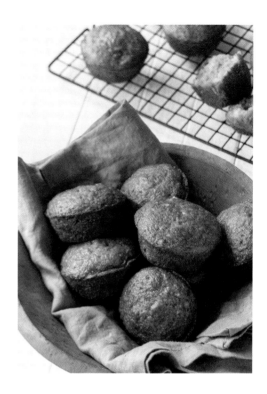

2 cups gluten-free all-purpose flour
1 cup plain organic cornmeal
2 teaspoons baking soda
½ teaspoon salt
2 cups plain yogurt
1 cup agave nectar
½ cup extra-virgin oil
2 teaspoons orange zest
1 teaspoon pure vanilla extract
1 cup chopped dried fruit

1. Preheat the oven to 350 degrees.
2. Line 16 muffin cups with paper liners and set aside.
3. In a large mixing bowl, stir together the flour, cornmeal, baking soda, and salt.
4. In a separate bowl, whisk together the yogurt, agave nectar, oil, orange zest, and extract.
5. Add to the flour mixture, stirring just until blended.
6. Fold in the dried fruit and evenly divide the batter among the muffin cups, filling no more than two-thirds full.
7. Bake for 24-27 minutes or until a cake tester inserted in the center comes out clean. The tops will be golden brown.
8. Let cool in the pan 2 minutes before transferring to a wire rack to cool completely.

One Pan Roasted Chicken & Garden Vegetable
Yield: 2 servings

This is a one-dish dinner for convenience and a great way to utilize any lingering vegetables from your own garden or the market. It can be prepped ahead of time, then just popped in the oven when you get home.

> 4 boneless, skinless chicken thighs
> 2 carrots, peeled and thickly sliced
> 1 zucchini, thickly sliced
> 1 yellow squash, thickly sliced
> 1 red onion, peeled and cut in wedges
> 3 tablespoons extra-virgin oil
> Juice of 1 lemon
> 2 tablespoons chopped fresh oregano
> 2 garlic cloves, peeled and minced
> ½ teaspoon salt
> ¼ teaspoon black pepper
> 12 cherry tomatoes
> Fresh parsley leaves for garnish

1. Preheat the oven to 400 degrees.
2. Coat a large rimmed baking dish with cooking spray and add the chicken, carrots, zucchini, squash, and onion wedges.
3. Place in as much of a single layer as possible.
4. In a small bowl, whisk together the oil, lemon juice, oregano, garlic, salt, and pepper. Pour over the chicken and vegetables.
5. Bake for 20 minutes.
6. Remove from the oven and scatter the tomatoes over the top.
7. Bake 15 minutes longer or until the chicken is cooked through.
8. Serve warm with a garnish of parsley.

Tomato Lentil Soup
Yield: 4 servings

This is a soup that you'll make on a regular basis because it's just the right mix of soothing, satisfying ingredients. You will love the flavor intensity it gets from the sun-dried tomatoes.

> 3 garlic cloves, peeled and minced
> 3 large carrots, peeled and coarsely grated
> 3 cups lentils
> 3 cups low sodium vegetable stock or water (see page 96)
> 3½ cups chopped tomatoes
> 1 (6-ounce) jar sun-dried tomatoes, packed in olive oil, drained and chopped
> 1 (6-ounce) can tomato paste
> 1 (8-ounce) package baby spinach
> 1 (15-ounce) can garbanzo beans, drained and rinsed
> ½ teaspoon onion or garlic salt
> ¼ teaspoon black pepper
> ¼ teaspoon crushed red pepper

1. Place the garlic, carrots, lentils, stock, chopped tomatoes, dried tomatoes, and tomato paste in a Dutch oven.
2. Place over medium high heat and bring to a boil.
3. Reduce the heat to simmer, cover, and cook for 45 minutes.
4. Stir in the spinach, garbanzo beans, salt, black pepper, and crushed red pepper.
5. Cook uncovered for 15 minutes longer and serve warm.

GREEN GOODNESS TABBOULEH
Yield: 3 servings

Bulgur wheat is more readily available than ever before. There was a time this wasn't the case! You can find it in several different grinds from fine to coarse, so use your preference. This tabbouleh is loaded with so much fresh green goodness from the herb garden that it becomes a great side salad.

1 cup bulgur wheat
1 large shallot, peeled and finely
    chopped
1 cup chopped fresh parsley
2 tablespoons chopped fresh mint
2 tablespoons extra-virgin oil
2 tablespoons lemon juice
½ teaspoon salt
¼ teaspoon black pepper

1. Bring 1¼ cups of water to a boil in a medium saucepan over high heat.
2. Stir in the bulgur wheat and immediately remove from the heat.
3. Cover and set aside for 20 minutes or until all the liquid has been absorbed.
4. Transfer to a serving bowl and stir in the chopped shallot pieces. Set aside to cool for 30 minutes.
5. Stir in the parsley, mint, oil, juice, salt, and pepper.
6. Serve immediately or refrigerate for later use. Bring to room temperature before serving.

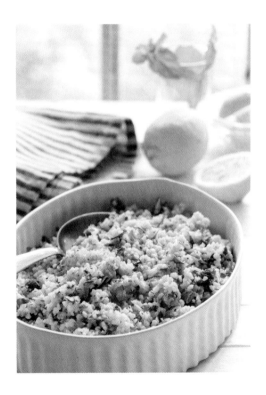

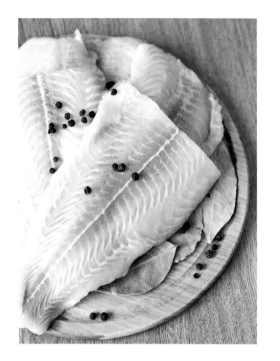

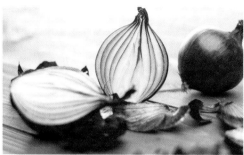

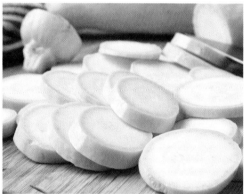

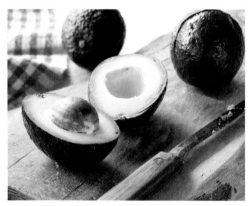

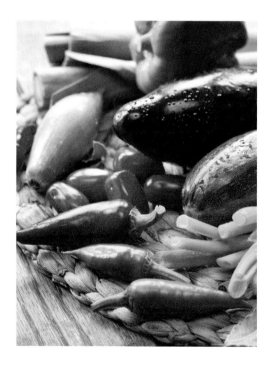

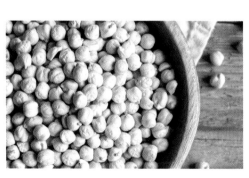

DAY 9

Homemade Low Sodium Chicken Stock
Yield: 7 cups

This stock uses the same formula for vegetable stock but customizes the vegetables and adds chicken bones. Save herbs, celery, carrots, and any type of onion scraps in the freezer for this concoction. The process is the same, but the result is very different. Each has a purpose and couldn't be easier to make.

Carcass from a roasted chicken
2 cups frozen vegetable scraps
7 cups water
2 bay leaves
1 teaspoon black peppercorns
½ teaspoon salt

1. Place the bones and vegetable scraps in a large slow cooker.
2. Add the water, bay leaves, peppercorns, and salt.
3. Cover and cook on low for 8 hours or on high for 4 hours.
4. Cool completely and strain with a fine mesh sieve. Discard solids.
5. Refrigerate and use within 4 days or package into freezer containers and freeze.

FOOD FACTS: CHICKEN

Read the label: Whole chickens labeled "broiler/fryer" weigh up to 3½ pounds and are typically less than three months old. Chickens labeled "roaster" have a higher fat content, can be up to 5 pounds, and are up to eight months old.

Unfried Fish
Yield: 2 servings

Baked fish simply doesn't have the same appeal as fried because the crunch is missing. This baked version with panko satisfies the crunch factor without the fat factor!

1 egg
1 tablespoon almond or coconut milk
1 cup panko, whole wheat, or
    gluten-free breadcrumbs
1 teaspoon dried dill
1 teaspoon dried parsley
2 fish fillets

1. Preheat the oven to 450 degrees and line a baking sheet with parchment. Set aside.

2. In a shallow dish, whisk together the egg and milk.
3. In a separate shallow dish, combine the panko, dill, and parsley.
4. Dip the fillets in the egg mixture then dredge them in the seasoned breadcrumbs.
5. Place on the baking sheet, pressing the breadcrumbs into the fish if necessary.
6. Bake 10 minutes or until the fish is completely done in the middle.
7. Allow to cool 5 minutes on the pan before serving warm.

FOOD FACT: TURKEY

Turkey tenderloins are sections of turkey breast meat that are low in fat and cook quickly.

SPICY SWEET TURKEY SOUP
Yield: 6 servings

You can turn this soup into a stew by decreasing the amount of stock used. It is just as delicious with boneless, skinless chicken.

2 tablespoons extra-virgin oil
1½ pounds turkey loin, cut into cubes
4 carrots, peeled and sliced
2 zucchini or summer squash, halved and sliced
2 garlic cloves, peeled and minced
1 sweet onion, peeled and coarsely chopped
2 tablespoons chili powder
2 teaspoons firmly packed light brown sugar
⅛ teaspoon black pepper
⅛ teaspoon ground ginger
⅛ teaspoon ground nutmeg
2 cups diced tomatoes (seeded if desired)
2 cups low sodium chicken stock (see page 117)
¼ cup apple cider vinegar
1 (15-ounce) can garbanzo or white beans, drained and rinsed
¼ cup chopped fresh parsley

1. Place the oil in a Dutch oven over medium-high heat.
2. When hot, add the turkey and sauté for 5 minutes, stirring frequently to brown on all sides.
3. Add the carrots, zucchini, garlic, and chopped onion pieces. Reduce the heat to medium and cook, stirring occasionally, for 5 minutes.
4. Stir in the chili powder, sugar, pepper, ginger, and nutmeg and cook 2 minutes longer, stirring frequently.
5. Increase the heat to high and add the diced tomato pieces, stock, and vinegar.
6. Bring to a boil, reduce the heat to low, cover, and simmer 30 minutes.
7. Uncover and stir in the beans.
8. Cook 3 minutes longer and serve warm with a garnish of chopped parsley.

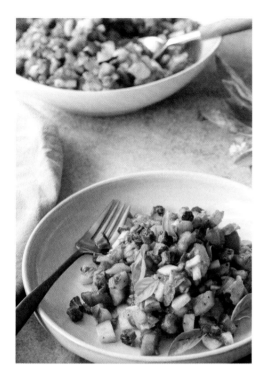

LATE HARVEST RATATOUILLE
Yield: 4 servings

This is a terrific way to put all those end-of-the-season vegetables to good use in a delicious stew. Top with some toasted whole wheat or gluten-free panko as a garnish.

2 tablespoons extra-virgin oil
1 sweet onion, peeled and chopped
1 large garlic clove, peeled and minced
1 large eggplant, peeled and cubed
2 small zucchini, chopped
4 tomatoes, diced (seeded if desired)
2 tablespoons tomato paste
⅓ cup water
¼ teaspoon black pepper
⅛ teaspoon cayenne
3 tablespoons chopped fresh parsley
Fresh basil sprigs for garnish

1. Place the oil in a large saucepan over high heat.
2. Add the chopped onion pieces and garlic and cook, stirring constantly for 1 minute.
3. Add the eggplant and reduce the heat to medium. Cook 5 minutes, stirring occasionally.
4. Add the zucchini and cook 2 minutes longer, stirring occasionally.
5. Stir in the tomatoes, tomato paste, water, black pepper, and cayenne. Bring to a simmer, cover, and cook for 8-10 minutes.
6. Remove from the heat, uncover, and let stand for 3 minutes.
7. Stir in the parsley, garnish with the basil, and serve warm.

FOOD FACT: SQUASH (SUMMER)

Size: While small to medium summer squash is perfect for grilling or sautéing, the larger ones are a little more of a challenge. And if you've ever grown squash, you'll certainly find one that has been hiding underneath the leaves and is huge. Those are the ones to shred or chop and roast or utilize in a baked product.

Gazpacho Salad
Yield: 2 servings

This is all the fresh goodness of gazpacho without the liquid. It benefits from sitting in the refrigerator for some time—if you can resist it that long!

1 orange bell pepper, seeded and chopped

1 cucumber, peeled, seeded, and chopped

1 large tomato, seeded and chopped

1 green onion, chopped

2 garlic cloves, peeled and minced

1 tablespoon chopped fresh basil

1 tablespoon chopped fresh parsley

2 tablespoons extra-virgin oil

1 tablespoon red wine, balsamic, or apple cider vinegar

½ teaspoon seasoned salt

¼ teaspoon black pepper

Baby spinach leaves

1. In a mixing bowl, combine the chopped bell pepper, cucumber, tomato, and onion pieces, garlic, basil, and parsley.
2. Drizzle with the oil and vinegar and sprinkle with the salt and pepper. Toss to evenly coat.
3. Cover and refrigerate at least 1 hour.
4. Serve cold or at room temperature on a bed of baby spinach leaves.

FOOD FACT: AVOCADOS

Selection: You will likely find rock hard avocados on the market, and they will take four to six days to soften when stored at room temperature. If they become too soft too quickly, place them in the refrigerator to slow down the process.

Edamame Guacamole
Yield: 6 servings

Bright green shelled soybeans (edamame) give this spread a nice texture. It can be a sandwich spread to replace mayonnaise or a great smear for raw veggies.

1 (16-ounce) package organic shelled edamame (if frozen, thawed)

1 avocado, halved, peeled, and pitted

1-2 tablespoons lemon juice

1-2 tablespoons extra-virgin oil

¼ teaspoon white pepper

¼ teaspoon hot sauce

1. Place the edamame, avocadoes, lemon juice, oil, pepper, and hot sauce in the bowl of a food processor. Puree until smooth.
2. If necessary, add a tablespoon of water to make the mixture smoother.
3. Serve with carrot sticks, celery sticks, cauliflower or broccoli florets, or baked tortilla chips (see page 125).

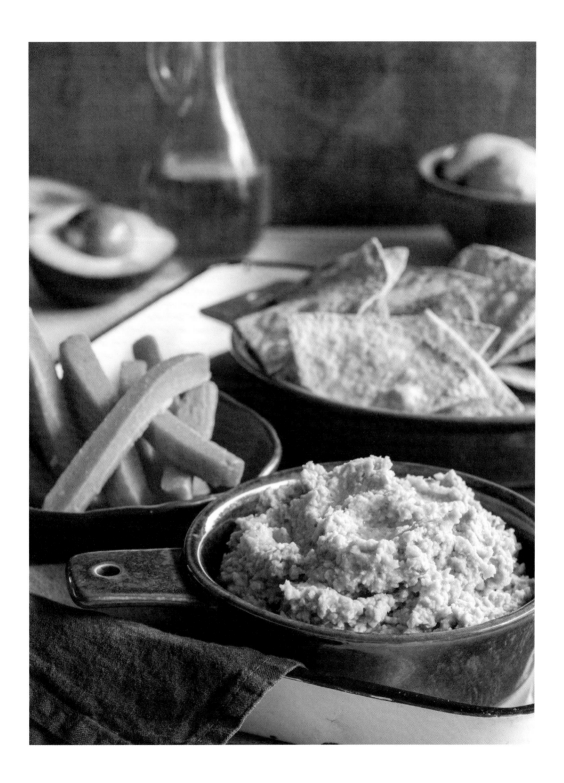

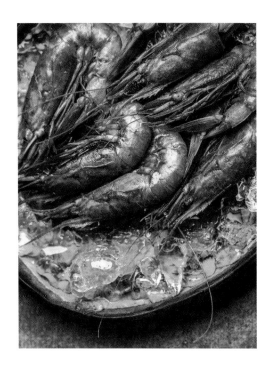

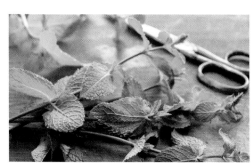

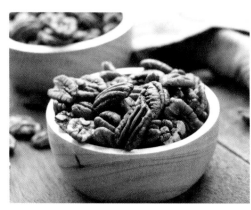

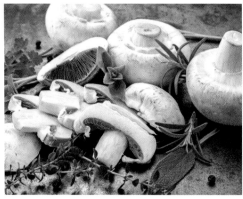

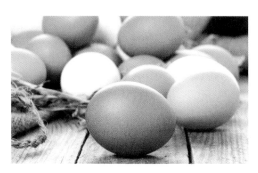

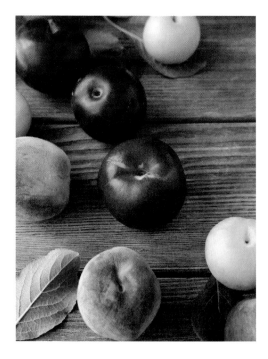

DAY 10

BUCK WHEAT PANCAKES
Yield: 2 servings

Yes, you can enjoy pancakes while following this modified Mediterranean Diet, and this buck wheat version is as light and fluffy as it gets. Be careful not to over mix the batter! Serve with fresh fruit or saute 1 tablespoon to ¼ cup of fruit in grass-fed butter to make your own delicious syrup.

  ¾ cup buck wheat flour
  1 teaspoon baking powder
  ⅛ teaspoon salt
  ¾ cup almond or coconut milk
  1 egg

1. Preheat the oven to 200 degrees.
2. In a mixing bowl, combine the flour, baking powder, and salt.
3. In a separate bowl, whisk together the milk and egg.
4. Pour into the flour mixture and stir just until combined.
5. Lightly coat a griddle with cooking spray and place over medium heat.
6. Ladle the batter into the warm pan and allow bubbles to form around the edges.
7. Flip and cook another 2 or 3 minutes.
8. Repeat with the remaining batter. Serve warm.

GRILLED CITRUS SHRIMP
Yield: 2 servings

Marinating the shrimp for just an hour in the refrigerator makes all the difference in the world to this dish. Serve it over Boston lettuce with a mixture of chopped yellow, red, and orange bell peppers and a sprinkling of black beans and fresh cilantro.

  1 lime or lemon
  2 garlic cloves, peeled and minced
  1 tablespoon extra-virgin olive oil
  1 teaspoon sesame oil
  ¼ teaspoon ground cumin
  ¼ teaspoon black pepper
  1 pound large shrimp, peeled and
    deveined with tails attached
  1 teaspoon chopped fresh cilantro

1. Cut the lime in half and squeeze the juice from one half into a small bowl.
2. Add the garlic, olive oil, sesame oil, cumin, and pepper to the lime juice and whisk.
3. Place the shrimp in a zip-top bag and add the marinade, shaking to thoroughly coat. Seal and refrigerate at least 1 hour.
4. Meanwhile, cut the remaining lime in half and then into thick slices. Set aside.

5. Preheat the grill to medium-high and thread the shrimp on skewers with the lime slices.
6. Cook about 3 minutes on each side or until the shrimp turn bright pink.
7. Transfer to a serving plate and garnish with the cilantro. Serve warm.

Mushroom & Pearl Barley Stuffing
Yield: 6 servings

Don't relegate stuffing just to the holiday season! It is a great low carb alternative to traditional stuffing and dressing and can be enjoyed alongside a variety of main dishes.

1 (1-ounce) package dried porcini mushrooms
2 cups hot water
2 tablespoons extra-virgin oil
1 (8-ounce) package sliced mushrooms
2 celery stalks, chopped
2 garlic cloves, peeled and minced
1 sweet onion, peeled and chopped
½ teaspoon dried oregano
½ teaspoon dried thyme
½ teaspoon salt
¼ teaspoon black pepper
2 cups pearl barley
3 cups low sodium organic chicken stock (see page 117)
3 tablespoons chia seeds
2 tablespoons grated Parmesan cheese

1. Place the dried mushrooms in a bowl and add the hot water. Set aside for 20 minutes to rehydrate.
2. Use a slotted spoon to remove the mushrooms and coarsely chop. Reserve the soaking liquid.
3. Place the oil in a large saucepan over medium-high heat.
4. When hot, add the sliced mushrooms, celery, garlic, chopped onion pieces, oregano, thyme, salt, and pepper. Cook 10 minutes.
5. Meanwhile, preheat the oven to 400 degrees.
6. Lightly grease a 3-quart baking dish with cooking spray and set aside.
7. Add the chopped porcini mushrooms and barley to the saucepan. Cook stirring frequently for 4 minutes.
8. Add the stock and reserved soaking liquid and bring to a boil. Remove from the heat and stir in the chia seeds and cheese.
9. Transfer to the prepared baking dish and bake for 40 minutes. Serve warm.

FOOD FACT: CELERY

Selection: Choose firm bunches that are tight. The leaves at the top should be bright green and the entire bunch should be crisp.

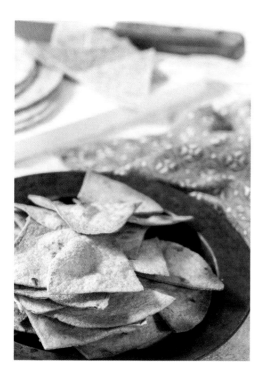

3. Add the tortilla wedges to the pan in a single layer. Spray the tops with more cooking spray.
4. Bake 7 to 9 minutes or until light golden brown.
5. Remove from the pan and cool on a wire rack. Serve warm or at room temperature.

FOOD FACT: HERBS

Storage: Washed herbs that you will be using shortly can be wrapped in a paper towel and placed in the refrigerator. If you cut more than you can use right away, treat them as you would fresh cut flowers. Place them in a vase with a couple of inches of water. Refrigerate, and if you don't use within a couple of days, change the water and cut the ends.

BAKED TORTILLA CHIPS
Yield: 2 servings

The trusty oven comes to the rescue once more because, in case you haven't heard, fried is out and baked is in! That goes for these tortilla chips, as well as other foods. The crunch doesn't go away, but the extra fat does!

    2 (8-inch) gluten-free, whole wheat, or
        organic corn tortillas, cut into
        8 wedges

1. Preheat the oven to 350 degrees.
2. Lightly grease a cookie sheet with cooking spray.

CURED MINTED FRUIT
Yield: 2-3 servings

The natural flavors that come to the surface when stone fruits are drizzled with just a bit of vinegar will blow your mind. And since all of these fruits hit the market at the same time, it's easy to turn this into a regular summer snack or dessert. It is just as nice with one of the fruits if you have extra.

2 plums, pitted and sliced

1 large peach, peeled, pitted and
    sliced

1 nectarine, pitted and sliced

1 tablespoon balsamic vinegar

Chopped fresh mint for garnish

1. Place the plum, peach and nectarine
   slices in a shallow bowl and drizzle with
   the vinegar. Cover and allow to stand
   for at least 30 minutes.
2. Garnish with the mint and serve.

NUTTY BAKED CATFISH
Yield: 2 servings

Leave it to nuts to add just the right amount
of crunch to oven baked catfish. You can
utilize any nut you wish, from pecans to
walnuts to cashews, and you can change up
the fish for variety as well. Finely chopping
the nuts in the food processor gives you the
best results.

¼ cup almond, coconut, or low fat milk

¼ teaspoon black pepper

¼ teaspoon cayenne

2 catfish fillets

1 cup nuts

1 garlic clove, peeled

⅓ cup panko, whole wheat, or
    gluten-free breadcrumbs

Fresh parsley sprigs for garnish

1. Preheat the oven to 375 degrees.
2. Place the milk, pepper, and cayenne
   in a shallow dish and add the fillets.
   Let soak 5 minutes, then turn.
3. Line a baking sheet with parchment
   paper, lightly grease and set aside.
4. Place the nuts, garlic, and panko in
   the bowl of a food processor and pulse
   to grind.
5. Remove the fillets from the milk bath
   and transfer to the prepared baking
   sheet.
6. Top evenly with the breadcrumb
   mixture, mashing slightly to adhere.
7. Bake 20 minutes or until the fish flakes
   easily with a fork.
8. Let rest for 5 minutes and serve warm
   with a garnish of parsley.

FOOD FACT: FISH

Catfish gets its name from the
whisker-like barbels that hang
down from the mouth area. These
are actually feelers. The fish is firm,
but mild in taste, so feel free to
enhance it with fresh herbs.

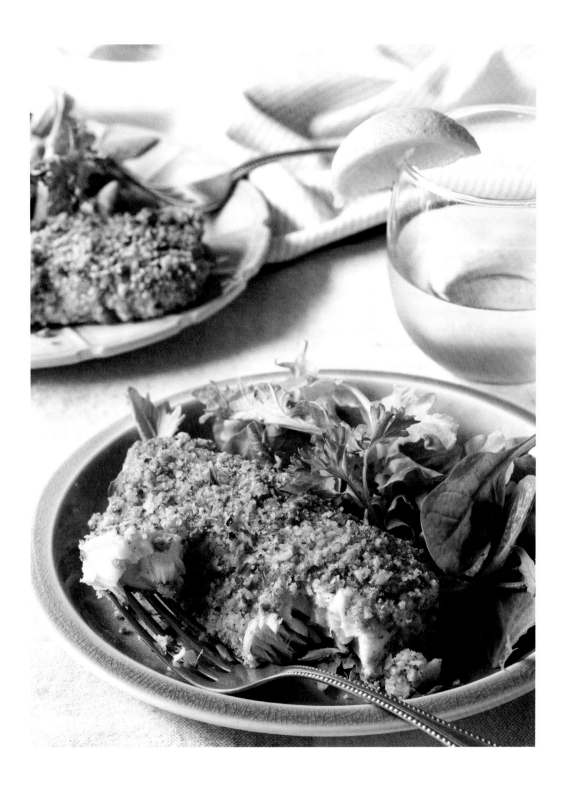

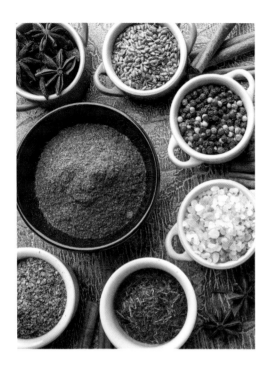

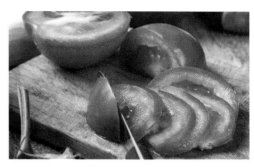

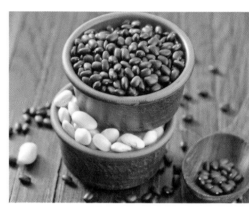

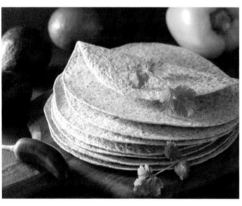

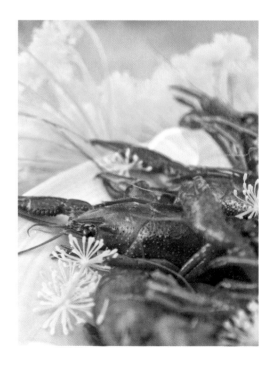

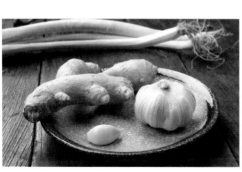

DAY 11

SPICED GINGER MUFFINS
Yield: about 16 muffins

This is a symphony of noticeable ginger accompanied by allspice, cinnamon, and cloves. If you can't find sorghum syrup, substitute with molasses or honey.

2½ cup gluten-free flour
1 tablespoon ground ginger
1½ teaspoons baking soda
1¼ teaspoons ground cinnamon
½ teaspoon ground allspice
½ teaspoon salt
¼ teaspoon ground cloves
1 cup sorghum syrup
2 teaspoons apple cider vinegar
1 cup boiling water
½ cup firmly packed light brown sugar
½ cup extra-virgin oil
2 teaspoons pure vanilla extract

1. Preheat the oven to 375 degrees.
2. Line 16 muffin cups with paper liners and set aside.
3. In a mixing bowl, stir together the all-purpose flour, whole wheat flour, ginger, baking soda, cinnamon, allspice, salt, and cloves.
4. In a 4-cup glass measuring cup, combine the sorghum and vinegar.
5. Stir in the boiling water with the sorghum and vinegar. Allow to stand.
6. Meanwhile add the brown sugar, oil, and extract to the flour mixture.
7. Stir until well blended then slowly add the sorghum mixture, stirring until just blended.
8. Divide the batter evenly among the muffin cups, filling no more than two-thirds full.
9. Bake for 22-26 minutes or until a cake tester inserted in the center comes out clean.
10. Let cool 2 minutes in the pan, then transfer to a wire rack to cool completely.

FOOD FACT: WHOLE WHEAT FLOUR

Storage: Not all flours are the same, and the higher fat content of whole wheat flour makes it necessary to store it in the refrigerator. Make sure it's kept in an air-tight container so it doesn't absorb odors from other foods.

Black Bean & Crawfish Tacos
Yield: 2 servings

This unique combination works thanks to the sweet crawfish paired with spiced black beans. It is especially nice in the spring and early summer when the crawfish season is in full gear.

> 1 (15.5-ounce) can black beans, drained and rinsed
> 1 teaspoon paprika
> ½ teaspoon garlic powder
> ½ teaspoon cayenne
> ¼ teaspoon black pepper
> 2 cups cooked crawfish
> 4 whole wheat, gluten-free, or organic corn tortillas
> 1 large tomato, seeded and chopped
> ¼ cup plain Greek yogurt for garnish

1. Place the beans in a glass bowl and stir in the paprika, garlic powder, cayenne, and pepper.
2. Cover and microwave for 1 minute.
3. Stir and add the crawfish.
4. Cover and microwave 15 seconds longer. Keep covered and set aside.
5. Wrap the tortillas in a slightly damp dish towel and place in a covered dish.
6. Microwave for 20 seconds.
7. Uncover and add the black bean and crawfish mixture to the warm tortillas. Top with the chopped tomato pieces and drizzle with the yogurt. Serve warm.

FOOD FACT: TOMATOES

Storage: Go near the refrigerator with a fresh uncut tomato and you'll have summer reruns of how tomatoes taste during the winter months. Refrigerators and tomatoes do not like each other, so just don't do it! The only time a tomato should be refrigerated is if you have cut leftovers. Whole ones stay on the kitchen counter at room temperature.

White & Black Bean Soup
Yield: 6 servings

This deeply flavorful soup is a nice mix of fresh ingredients and convenient canned beans. You can use dried beans instead of canned, cooked per the recipe found on page 95.

> 2 tablespoons extra-virgin oil
> 1 sweet onion, peeled and chopped
> 3 garlic cloves, peeled and minced
> 2 carrots, peeled and sliced
> 2 celery stalks, chopped
> 4 cups low sodium, organic vegetable or chicken stock (see page 96 or 117)
> 3½ cups diced tomatoes
> 2 (15.5-ounce) cans black beans, drained and rinsed
> 1 (15.5-ounce) can white or Northern beans, drained and rinsed

2 tablespoons red wine or apple cider
    vinegar
1½ tablespoons chili powder
1 tablespoon dried basil
½ teaspoon salt
¼ teaspoon black pepper
¼ teaspoon crushed red pepper

1. Place the oil in a Dutch oven over
   medium heat.
2. When hot, add the chopped onion
   pieces and garlic. Cook, stirring
   frequently for 3 minutes.
3. Add the carrots and celery and cook
   3 minutes longer.
4. Stir in the stock and tomatoes and bring
   to a boil. Reduce the heat to low and
   simmer uncovered for 10 minutes.
5. Meanwhile, puree one can of the black
   beans in a food processor until smooth.
6. Add to the soup, along with the
   remaining can of black beans, white
   beans, vinegar, chili powder, basil, salt,
   black pepper, and crushed red pepper.
7. Cover and cook 15 minutes longer.
   Serve warm.

FRESH TOMATO COULIS
Yield: about 2 cups

This should be named "Use for Everything
Sauce" because it's that versatile. It can be a
vegetable dip, a sauce for spaghetti squash
noodles, poured over grilled meat, or even
as a salad dressing. Get to know it by using it
as a dip for mushrooms and go from there!

3 large tomatoes, seeded, peeled,
    and pureed
2 tablespoons chopped fresh basil
2 tablespoons balsamic vinegar
2 tablespoons extra-virgin oil
2 teaspoons tomato paste
½ teaspoon saffron threads
½ teaspoon garlic salt
¼ teaspoon black pepper

1. In a mixing bowl, whisk together the
   tomato puree, vinegar, oil, tomato paste,
   saffron, salt, and pepper.
2. Vigorously whisk for 1 minute to
   thoroughly blend.
3. Use immediately or cover and refrigerate
   for later use.

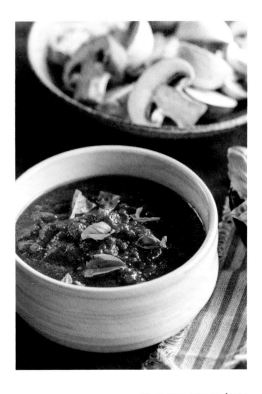

3. Process until the mixture just begins to come together.
4. Roll into balls and place on a baking sheet lined with waxed paper.
5. Refrigerate at least 2 hours before serving.

DRIED FRUIT BALLS
Yield: around 18 balls

The only problem with this snack is that it can test your patience. There's no baking necessary . . . you just need a food processor and a couple of hours in the refrigerator for them to firm up a bit—if you can wait that long!

  ½ cup pine nuts
  ½ cup dried pineapple
  ½ cup unsweetened shredded
      coconut
  ¼ cup dried cherries or dried
      cranberries
  2 tablespoons coconut oil, melted

1. Place the pine nuts in a food processor and pulse to make a flour.
2. Add the pineapple, coconut, cherries or cranberries, and oil.

SWEET POTATO HASH BROWNS
Yield: 2 servings

While some think potatoes must be shredded for hash browns, these are diced and water blanched. You can do those steps ahead if necessary.

  1 large sweet potato, peeled
      and diced
  2 tablespoons sorghum or maple
      syrup
  ½ teaspoon salt
  ¼ teaspoon black pepper
  3 tablespoons extra-virgin oil
  1 small sweet onion, peeled,
      and diced

1. Bring a large saucepan of water to a boil over high heat.
2. Add the sweet potatoes and blanch for 2 minutes. Drain and plunge into ice cold water. Immediately drain well and transfer to a medium bowl.

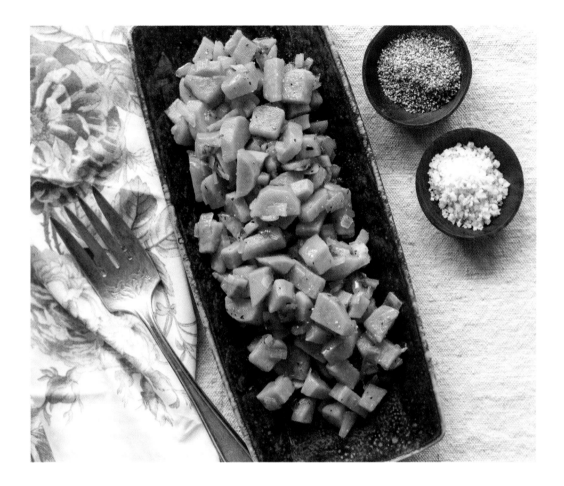

3. Add the syrup, salt, and pepper, tossing gently. Refrigerate for 15 to 20 minutes

4. Place the oil in a large sauté pan over medium-high heat.

5. When warm, add the diced onion pieces and cook for 5 minutes.

6. Stir in the sweet potatoes and any juices. Sauté 15 to 17 minutes, stirring gently and occasionally.

7. When golden brown, serve warm.

FOOD FACT: SWEET POTATOES

Curing: Early season sweet potatoes are "green" or uncured. These have a relatively short storage life, so buy them in small amounts and plan to use them soon. Late season sweet potatoes are cured by keeping them at controlled temperatures, which increases the shelf life.

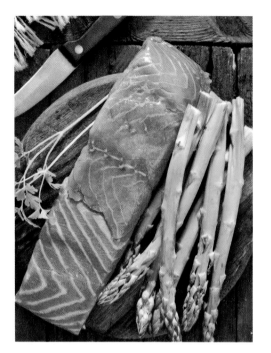
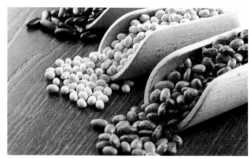
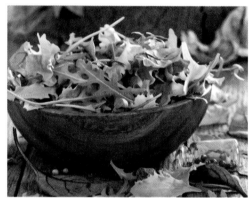
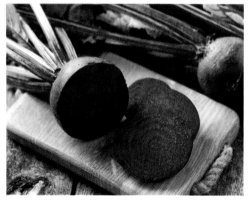
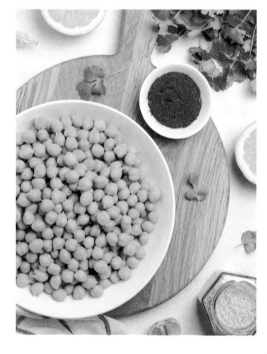
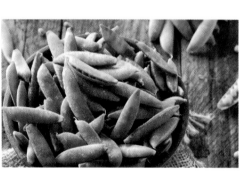

DAY 12

Beet & Cashew Slaw
Yield: 3 to 4 servings

Beets are not for everyone, but this recipe might change reluctant minds. It is hard to stop nibbling on it!

3 beets
4 carrots, peeled and cut into
    matchsticks
1 English cucumber, cut into
    matchsticks
3 tablespoons buttermilk
1½ teaspoons apple cider vinegar
½ teaspoon stevia
½ teaspoon salt
¼ teaspoon black pepper
⅓ cup cashews, chopped and divided
1 tablespoon chopped fresh parsley

1. Place a saucepan of water over high heat and bring to a boil.
2. Add the beets and cook for 10 minutes.
3. Drain and rinse under cold water to remove the skins, then set aside to cool.
4. Meanwhile, place the carrots and cucumber sticks in a serving bowl.
5. In a separate bowl, whisk together the buttermilk, vinegar, stevia, salt, and pepper.
6. Cut the cooled beets into matchsticks and add to the carrot mixture.
7. Drizzle with the dressing and half of the cashews. Toss to gently coat.
8. Top with the remaining cashews and parsley and serve.

FOOD FACT: BEETS

Selection: Small is my preference for size and if the leafy tops are still attached, remove them as soon as you get home. They pull moisture from the root and will shorten the shelf life. Make sure the beets are hard.

Zesty Salmon Salad
Yield: 2 servings

All kinds of beautiful vegetables arrive to local markets in the late spring months and continue through the summer. And all of them come together in this exceptional fresh salad that showcases each item perfectly. Use whatever chopped fresh herbs you have springing up in your garden as an accent.

6 asparagus spears, trimmed
and cut in 1-inch pieces

2 cups sugar snap peas

1 pound skinless salmon fillets,
cut in large cubes

½ teaspoon onion salt

¼ teaspoon lemon pepper

6 cups chopped heart of romaine

2 small radishes, trimmed and sliced

1 tablespoon chopped fresh chives

1 tablespoon chopped fresh parsley

2 tablespoons extra-virgin oil

1 tablespoon white wine, champagne,
or apple cider vinegar

1. Preheat the broiler on high.
2. Bring a large saucepan of water to a boil over high heat.
3. Add the asparagus and sugar snap peas and cook 2 and ½ minutes.
4. Drain and run under cold water for 1 minute. Set aside to drain thoroughly.
5. Place the salmon on a greased broiler rack and sprinkle evenly with the salt and pepper.
6. Broil for 3 minutes or until the salmon is done. Set aside to cool slightly.
7. Place the romaine in a serving bowl and add the, radishes, chives, and parsley, along with the asparagus and peas.
8. Drizzle with the oil and vinegar and toss to evenly coat.
9. Serve immediately.

NOT FRIED REFRIED BEANS
Yield: 2 to 3 servings

Welcome to all the taste without the fat of traditional refried beans. Anything that is leftover can become a great sandwich spread. Spice it up as much as you like.

1 (15-ounce) can pinto beans, drained and rinsed

½ cup salsa (see page 187)

¼ teaspoon cayenne, or more if desired

1. Lightly coat the bottom of a saucepan with cooking spray.
2. Add the beans and crush with a potato masher.
3. Place over medium heat and add the salsa and cayenne.
4. After 5 minutes, mash again until the desired consistency is reached. Serve warm.

FOOD FACT: SALMON

Salmon are anadromous, which means they live in saltwater but spawn in fresh water. Farmed salmon are raised in saltwater and usually lack the characteristic flavor of those from the wild.

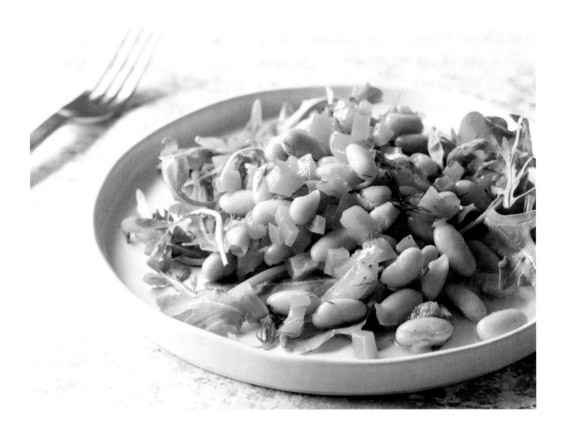

ARUGULA BEAN SALAD
Yield: 3 servings

Peppery arugula is calmed down with cannellini beans, then kicked back up with a fresh lemon vinaigrette. Because the beans are canned and ready to serve, the salad is ready to serve in an instant.

6 cups coarsely chopped arugula
1 (15.5-ounce) can cannellini or white beans, drained and rinsed
1 orange bell pepper, seeded and chopped

3 tablespoons extra-virgin oil
1½ tablespoons lemon juice
1 garlic clove, peeled and minced
1½ teaspoons chopped fresh dill
½ teaspoon salt
¼ teaspoon black pepper

1. Place the arugula, beans, and chopped bell pepper pieces in a serving bowl.
2. In a small bowl, whisk together the oil, juice, garlic, dill, salt, and pepper.
3. Add to the salad, tossing well to combine. Serve immediately.

SUMMER GAZPACHO
Yield: 6 servings

When you need to use up odds and ends in the vegetable crisper drawer, this is your go-to recipe. It is as much of a feast for the eyes as it is for your appetite!

- 4 cups low sodium tomato juice
- 3 cups diced tomatoes
- 4 green onions, trimmed and sliced
- 1 cucumber, peeled and diced
- 1 celery stalk, chopped
- 1 large yellow bell pepper, seeded and chopped
- 1 small sweet onion, peeled and chopped
- 2 garlic cloves, peeled and minced
- 3 tablespoons red wine or apple cider vinegar
- 1½ tablespoons extra-virgin oil
- ½ teaspoon stevia
- 1 teaspoon chopped fresh tarragon or basil
- ½ teaspoon salt
- ¼ teaspoon black pepper

1. In a large mixing bowl, stir together the juice, tomatoes, green onions, diced cucumber pieces, celery, chopped bell pepper and sweet onion pieces, and garlic.
2. In a small mixing bowl, whisk together the vinegar, oil, stevia, tarragon, salt, and pepper.
3. Stir into the soup, cover, and refrigerate at least 2 hours.
4. Serve room temperature or chilled.

TRADITIONAL HUMMUS
Yield: 4 servings

It's hard to beat this classic Mediterranean recipe. It is terrific as a raw vegetable dip as well as a sandwich spread that you can use to replace mayonnaise. Keep it in the refrigerator as a protein pick-up.

- 1 (15-ounce) can garbanzo beans (chickpeas), drained and rinsed
- 3 garlic cloves, peeled and minced
- 3 tablespoons lemon juice
- 2 tablespoons extra-virgin oil
- 1 teaspoon ground cumin
- ¼ teaspoon black pepper
- ¼ teaspoon hot sauce

1. Place the garbanzo beans, garlic, lemon juice, oil, cumin, pepper, and hot sauce in the bowl of a food processor. Puree until smooth.
2. Refrigerate up to 1 week.

Note: If you want the hummus to be a little smoother, add a tablespoon or two of water.

Roasted Red Pepper Variation:
1. Preheat the oven to 425 degrees. Slice a large red bell pepper into 8 long strips, discarding the seedy center.
2. Place on an ungreased baking sheet and roast for 10 minutes.
3. Cool and add to the food processor with the hummus recipe and 1 teaspoon of paprika.

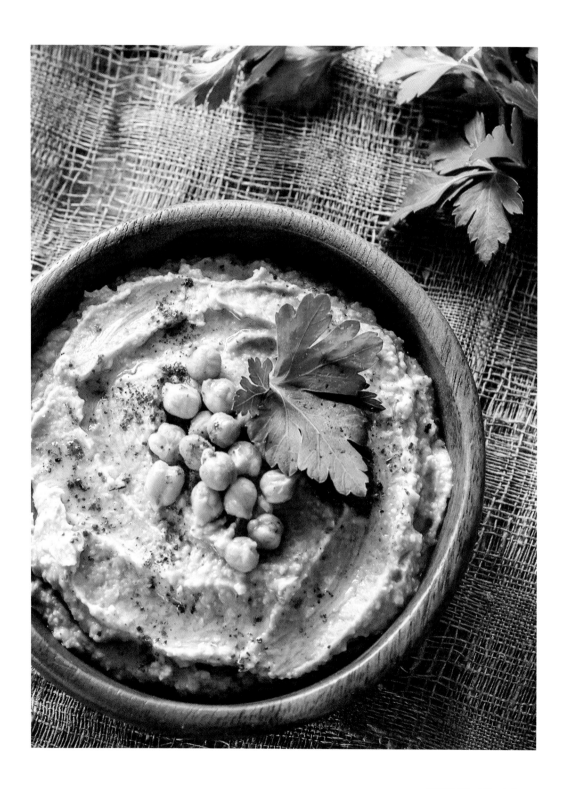

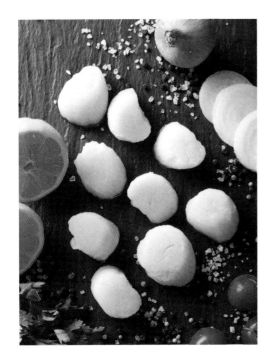
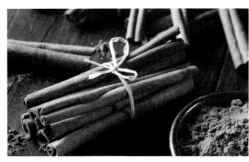
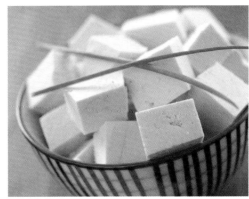
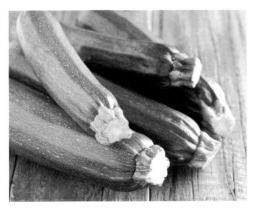
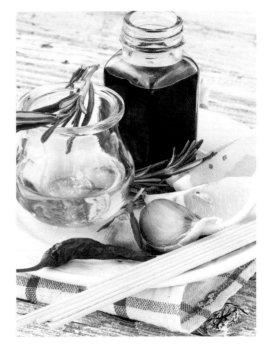
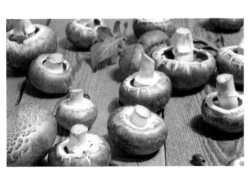

DAY 13

DRIED FRUIT COMPOTE
Yield: 6 servings

Dried fruits are flavor powerhouses. Here, they are rehydrated overnight so you've got a nice, soft texture. I like to use a mixture of dried apricots, golden raisins, apples, prunes, and cherries or cranberries. Serve this warm, room temperature, or cold.

  3 cups mixed unsweetened dried fruit
  4½ cups water, divided
  ¼ cup unsweetened pomegranate
      juice
  1 cinnamon stick
  ½ teaspoon lemon zest

1. Place the dried fruit in a large mixing bowl and add 3 cups of the water.
2. Cover and allow to stand overnight.
3. Drain the fruit, discarding the soaking liquid.
4. Transfer the fruit to a large saucepan and place over medium-low heat.
5. Add the remaining water, juice, cinnamon stick, and lemon zest.
6. Bring to a simmer then reduce the heat to low. Simmer 10 minutes.
7. Transfer the fruit to a serving bowl using a slotted spoon.
8. Continue to simmer the liquid for 25 minutes.
9. Remove and discard the cinnamon stick.
10. Pour the sauce over the fruit.
11. Serve immediately or cool and refrigerate for later use.

FOOD FACT: CITRUS

Freezing: Citrus zest and juice can be easily frozen for up to six months. Package the zest in the smallest container you can find. Juice can be frozen in pre-measured amounts in an ice cube tray, then transferred to a large zip-top freezer bag.

PLANTAIN LENTIL SALAD
Yield: 2 servings

Known as the "cooking banana," plantains are a fun way to add a bit of variety to your menus. Just about anything you do with a potato, you can do with a plantain. It has a thick skin and needs to be yellow with black splotches for this recipe. Leave it on the countertop at room temperature until ready.

1 ripe plantain

1¼ cups cooked lentils

1 large shallot, peeled and chopped

2 tablespoons red wine or apple cider
   vinegar

1 tablespoon extra-virgin oil

¼ teaspoon black pepper

¼ teaspoon paprika

Mixed salad greens

1. Preheat the oven to 450 degrees.
2. Cut the ends off the plantain and peel.
3. Cut into half-inch slices and place on a lightly greased baking sheet in a single layer.
4. Bake 12 to 15 minutes, turning halfway through.
5. In a medium bowl, combine the lentils, chopped shallot pieces, vinegar, oil, pepper, and paprika. Set aside.
6. When the plantains are golden and tender, remove from the oven and cool slightly.
7. Stir into the lentil mixture and serve on top of mixed salad greens.

FOOD FACT: HERBS

Washing: Freshly snipped herbs should be gently washed with a cool spray of water. Then shake the excess water from the leaves.

GRILLED SCALLOP & MUSHROOM PACKETS
Yield: 2 servings

Aluminum foil packets keep this special occasion treat from falling through the grill rack. They also keep everything moist and the servings divided. If you don't have herbs de provence, substitute a combination of rosemary and oregano or basil.

1 pound large scallops

1 (8-ounce) package whole
   mushrooms, washed

1 tablespoon extra-virgin oil

1 garlic clove, peeled and minced

1 tablespoon herbs de provence

¼ teaspoon garlic salt

Fresh parsley for garnish

1. Preheat the grill to medium-low.
2. Evenly divide the scallops and mushrooms onto large pieces of heavy-duty aluminum foil.
3. In a small bowl, stir together the oil, garlic, herbs de provence, and salt. Drizzle over the scallops and mushrooms.
4. Fold the foil into packets, making sure to seal the ends.
5. Place on the rack with the seam side up and grill 10 minutes.
6. Remove and let stand 5 minutes before unwrapping and serving with a garnish of fresh parsley.

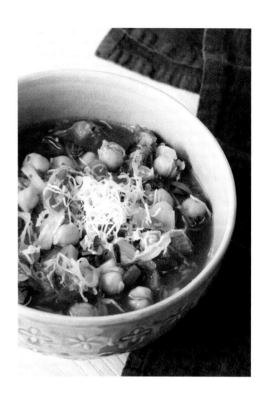

MINESTRONE SOUP WITH CHICKPEAS
Yield: 8 servings

Traditional minestrone soup is a thick vegetable soup that includes small, bite-sized pasta. This one substitutes chickpeas to give you the same look but with better sustenance. You won't miss the pasta! It makes a lot, so get your freezer containers ready for the excess.

1 tablespoon extra-virgin oil

2 large carrots, peeled and chopped

2 celery stalks, chopped

2 garlic cloves, peeled and minced

1 sweet onion, peeled and chopped

4 cups low sodium vegetable stock, divided (see page 96)

2 cups shredded cabbage

1 (15.5-ounce) can chickpeas, drained and rinsed

1 (14.5-ounce) can diced tomatoes, undrained

1 (8-ounce) can low sodium tomato sauce

1 tablespoon dried basil

2 teaspoon dried parsley

½ teaspoon dried oregano

½ teaspoon black pepper

¼ teaspoon dried thyme

¼ teaspoon paprika

1 cup chopped baby spinach

Grated Parmesan for garnish

1. Place the oil in a Dutch oven over medium-high heat.
2. When hot, add the carrots, celery, garlic, and chopped onion pieces.
3. Cook, stirring frequently for 2 minutes.
4. Stir in ½ cup of the stock and cook 5 minutes longer.

5. Add the remaining stock, cabbage, chickpeas, tomatoes, sauce, basil, parsley, oregano, pepper, thyme, and paprika.
6. Bring to a boil, cover, and reduce the heat to low. Simmer 25 minutes.
7. Stir in the spinach and remove from the heat.
8. Allow to stand covered for 5 minutes. Ladle into serving bowls and garnish with Parmesan.

Balsamic Glazed Zucchini
Yield: 2 servings

If you need a side dish in a hurry, this is your lucky recipe. It can be used for all types of soft-shelled summer squash, but try it first with prolific zucchini . . . a favorite!

    1 tablespoon extra-virgin oil
    2 zucchini, trimmed, halved and cut
        in ½-inch slices
    2 garlic cloves, peeled and minced
    ⅛ teaspoon salt
    Pinch of black pepper
    2 tablespoons balsamic vinegar
    2 teaspoons chopped fresh basil

1. Place the oil in a large skillet over high heat.
2. When hot, add the zucchini, stirring constantly for 1 minute.

3. Add the garlic, salt, and pepper and cook 2 minutes, or until the zucchini is evenly browned.
4. Stir in the vinegar and cook 1 minute to lightly glaze the zucchini.
5. Remove from the heat and add the basil. Serve warm.

FOOD FACT: SQUASH (SUMMER)

Since this squash is harvested while immature, the seeds are completely edible.

Glazed Tofu
Yield: 4 servings

If you think tofu is not for you, give this tremendous recipe a try. It can be a snack with whole wheat crackers or alone, or it can be a salad topping or even a wrap ingredient. You'll suddenly find loads of reasons to make it again!

    ¾ pound extra-firm organic tofu, drained
    2 tablespoons low sodium soy sauce
    2 tablespoons extra-virgin oil
    2 tablespoons pure maple syrup
    1 garlic clove, peeled and minced
    ½ teaspoon crushed red pepper

1. Place the tofu between paper towels and gently press to remove any excess water.
2. Place on a cutting board and cut into 4 slices. Set aside.
3. In a small bowl, whisk together the soy sauce, oil, syrup, garlic, and crushed red pepper.
4. Transfer sauce to a shallow sauté pan with a lid.
5. Place the tofu on top of the sauce in a single layer.
6. Place over high heat and bring the sauce mixture to a boil. Reduce the heat to medium, cover, and cook 4 minutes.
7. Flip the tofu and cook uncovered for 4 minutes longer.
8. Serve warm or at room temperature.

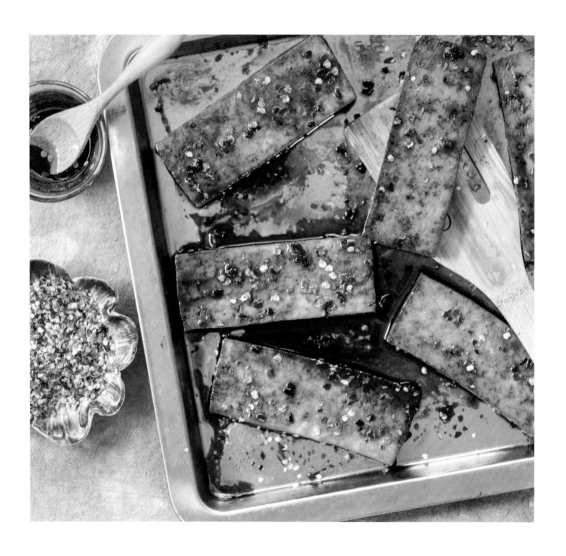

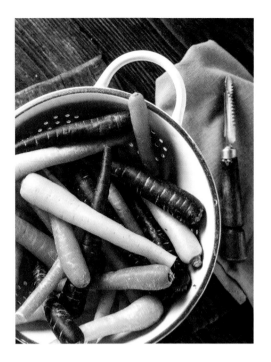
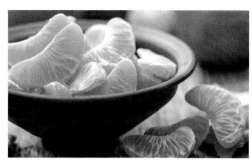
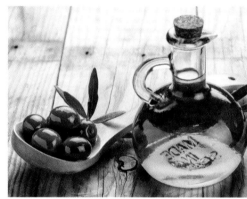
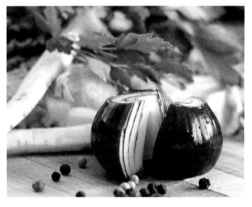
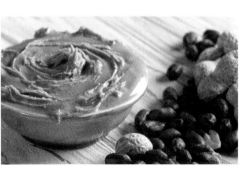
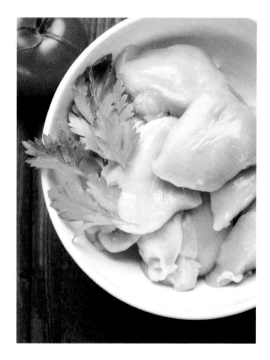

DAY 14

Date & Fig Morning Muffins
Yield: about 12 muffins

These muffins are beautifully dark and exceptionally moist. Make sure and use dried figs rather than fresh. This is another do-ahead recipe and requires a blender.

¾ cup chopped pitted dates

¾ cup chopped dried figs

1½ teaspoons baking soda

1 cup boiling water

1½ cup gluten-free all purpose flour

½ teaspoon baking powder

½ teaspoon salt

3 tablespoons ground flaxseeds

½ cup firmly packed light
    brown sugar

¼ cup extra-virgin oil

1 cup chopped walnuts

1. Place the dates, figs, and baking soda in a large mixing bowl and add the boiling water. Stir and allow to stand for 15 minutes.
2. Preheat the oven to 350 degrees.
3. Line 12 muffin cups with paper liners and set aside.
4. In a medium bowl, stir together the gluten-free flour, baking powder, and salt. Set aside.
5. Place the flaxseeds and ⅓ cup of water in a blender and process for 1 minute.
6. Add the sugar and oil and process another minute.
7. Pour into the date mixture and stir to combine.
8. Add the flour mixture and stir just until combined.
9. Fold in the walnuts.
10. Evenly divide the batter among the muffin cups, filling no more than two-thirds full.
11. Bake 20-23 minutes or until a cake tester inserted in the center comes out clean.
12. Let cool 3 minutes, then transfer to a wire rack to cool completely.

FOOD FACT: FLAXSEEDS

Grinding: It is much more economical to grind your own into meal. I simply place the seeds in a spice mill or coffee grinder and process until it is very fine.

Peanut Butter Spread
Yield: 1 cup

Smear this delightful spread on carrots, celery, and slices of bell peppers. Or thin with more hot tea and use it as a dip or a sauce for roasted veggies. Take your pick!

¾ cup hot brewed tea (black or green tea)
¼ teaspoon crushed red pepper
¾ cup natural peanut butter
2 green onions, thinly sliced
1 teaspoon low sodium soy sauce
Fresh cilantro for garnish

1. Measure 1 cup of the hot tea and add the crushed red pepper.
2. Allow to steep for 1 minute.
3. Meanwhile, place the peanut butter, onions, and soy sauce in a serving bowl.
4. Add the steeped tea and whisk until smooth.
5. Cool to room temperature or refrigerate for later use.
6. When ready to serve, bring to room temperature, garnish, and serve.

Granny's Sweet Potato Soup
Yield: 6 servings

The slow cooker comes to the rescue here and once cooked, allows this soup to be ready to enjoy in mere minutes. It is another great example of how soups can taste creamy without cream!

5 sweet potatoes, peeled and cut in chunks
2 Granny Smith apples, peeled, cored, and quartered
1 sweet onion, peeled and chopped
5½ cups low sodium, organic chicken stock (see page 117)
1 teaspoon chopped fresh thyme
¼ teaspoon white pepper
Fresh thyme for garnish

1. Place the sweet potatoes, apples, chopped onion pieces, stock, thyme, and pepper in a large slow cooker.
2. Cover and cook on low for 8 hours or on high for 4 hours.
3. Uncover and cool for 10 minutes.
4. With an immersion blender, puree the soup until smooth.
5. Garnish with fresh thyme and serve warm.

FOOD FACT: APPLES

Storage: Apples are just fine stored at room temperature. If you purchase them in bulk, go to the refrigerator. Place in a plastic bag with a couple of holes punched in it for air circulation. Add a tablespoon of water, close the bag and place in the crisper drawer.

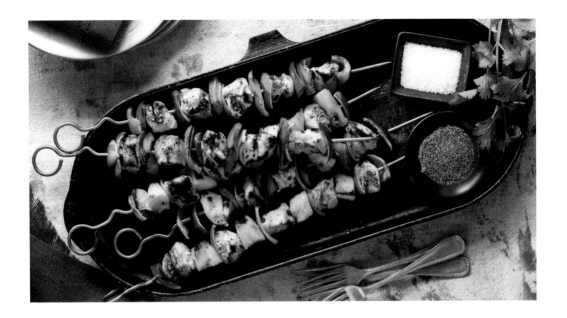

Tropical Chicken Kabobs
Yield: 2 servings

Using skewers can be a terrific way to control portion sizes. The fresh pineapple is what really takes this to a higher level. Substitute the fresh pineapple for brightly colored bell peppers if you wish.

2 garlic cloves, peeled and minced

1 tablespoon grated gingerroot

2 tablespoons lime juice

2 tablespoons extra-virgin oil

1 tablespoon raw honey

½ teaspoon crushed red pepper

2 cups of fresh pineapple, cut into 1-inch cubes

2 small boneless, skinless chicken breasts, cut in 1-inch cubes

1 small red onion, peeled and cut in wedges

1 tablespoon chopped fresh cilantro

1. In a jar with a tight-fitting lid, combine the garlic, gingerroot, lime juice, oil, honey, and crushed red pepper. Close and shake to emulsify.
2. Place the pineapple and chicken in a zip-top bag and add the garlic mixture. Close and refrigerate at least 2 hours.
3. Preheat the grill to medium-high.
4. Meanwhile, thread the pineapple, chicken, and onion wedges onto skewers, dividing evenly.
5. Grill 10 minutes, turning once and making sure the chicken is completely cooked.
6. Serve warm with a sprinkling of the cilantro.

NEW & IMPROVED CARROT SALAD
Yield: 2 servings

This is a far cry from the carrot raisin salad served at many family events. It has been improved by eliminating the heavy mayonnaise dressing and you will love the result.

   1 cup golden raisins
   2 cups boiling water
   1 (11-ounce) container mandarin
      orange slices, packed in juice
   4 carrots, peeled and slivered with
      a vegetable peeler
   1 cup pitted black or green olives
   1 teaspoon stevia
   1 teaspoon ground cumin
   ¼ teaspoon black pepper
   1½ cups whole cashews

1. Place the raisins in a medium glass measuring cup and add the boiling water. Set aside.

2. Place the oranges (drained)* in a serving bowl with the carrots and olives.
3. In a small skillet over medium heat, stir together 2 tablespoons of the reserved juice along with the stevia, cumin, and pepper.
4. Cook, stirring constantly for 1 minute, and add the cashews.
5. Cook 1 minute longer, stirring constantly.
6. Drain the raisins and add to the carrot mixture.
7. Drizzle with the cashew mixture, tossing well to coat.
8. If desired, add another tablespoon of the juice. Serve immediately.

*Note: Save the remaining juice from the mandarin oranges to use in smoothies.

SEARED HOMINY RELISH
Yield: 2 servings

Hominy is an interesting version of corn and can add lots of interest to a meal. You can add parsley if you desire, but don't leave out the cilantro!

   1 tablespoon extra-virgin oil
   1 (15.5-ounce) can golden hominy,
      drained and rinsed
   3 garlic cloves, peeled and minced

1 shallot, peeled and chopped

2 tomatoes, seeded and chopped

2 tablespoons red wine or apple cider vinegar

2 tablespoons extra-virgin oil

1 teaspoon chopped fresh cilantro

½ teaspoon salt

¼ teaspoon black pepper

1. Place the oil in a large sauté pan over high heat.

2. When hot, add the hominy and sear (without stirring) 2 minutes.

3. Toss well and sear another 2 minutes.

4. Add the garlic and chopped shallot pieces and sauté 2 minutes longer.

5. Remove from the heat and stir in the tomatoes, vinegar, olive oil, cilantro, salt, and pepper.

6. Toss well and serve warm or at room temperature.

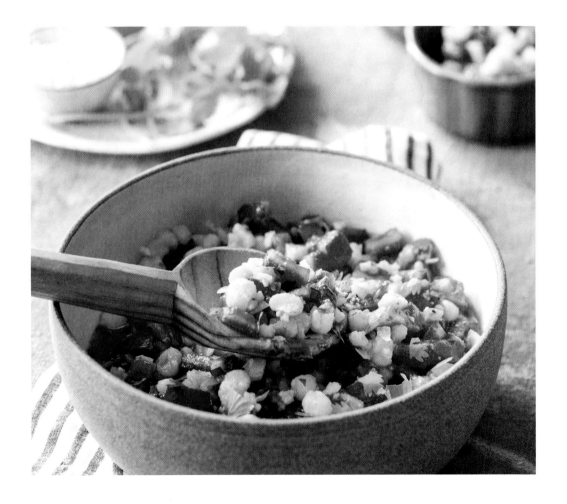

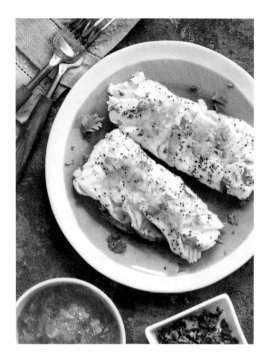

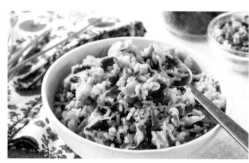

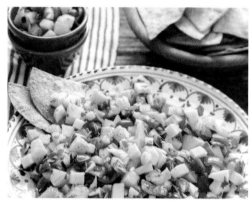

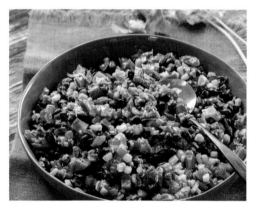

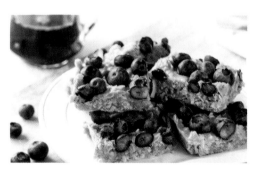

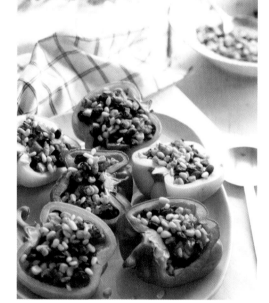

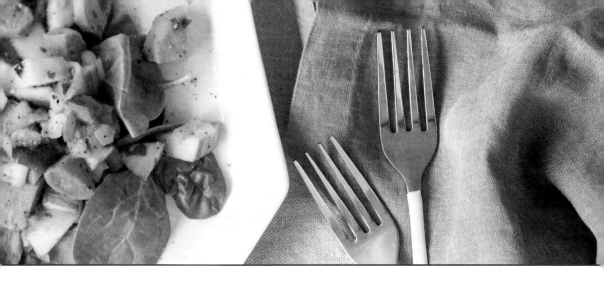

WEEK THREE

Days 15–21

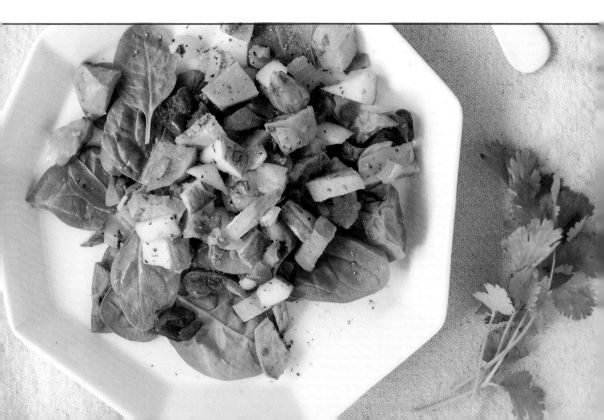

SHOPPING LIST – WEEK 3

(DAYS 15–21)

FRUIT

- ☐ Banana – 1
- ☐ Blackberries – 6-ounce container
- ☐ Blueberries – 6-ounce container
- ☐ Clementine or Tangerine – 1
- ☐ Grapefruit – 1
- ☐ Grapes – 1 small bunch
- ☐ Kiwi – 1
- ☐ Papaya or Mango – 1
- ☐ Pear or Pomegranate – 1
- ☐ Tangarine or Orange – 1
- ☐ Strawberries – 16-ounce container

VEGETABLES

- ☐ Asparagus – 3 bunches
- ☐ Broccoli – 7 day supply
- ☐ Cauliflower – 2 heads
- ☐ Corn – 1 ear
- ☐ Cucumbers – 7 day supply
- ☐ Eggplant – 2
- ☐ Green Beans – 7 day supply
- ☐ Leeks – 1 bunch
- ☐ Mushrooms – 7 day supply
- ☐ Okra – 1 serving size
- ☐ Pattypan or Yellow Squash – 2 medium
- ☐ Peppers (variety of colors) – 7 day supply
- ☐ Portabella Mushrooms – 2 large

- ☐ Salad Greens (chicory, spinach, kale, Belgian endive, bean sprouts, iceberg, romaine) – 7 day supply for twice daily salads
- ☐ Snow Peas – 1 serving size
- ☐ Turnip Greens or Bok Choy – 1 bunch
- ☐ Tomatillos – 3 (for salsa)
- ☐ Zucchini – 2 medium

MEAT

- ☐ Boneless, Skinless Chicken Breast*
- ☐ Catfish Fillet*
- ☐ Salmon Fillet*
- ☐ Shrimp (large)*
- ☐ Extra Lean Beef (96/4, petite fillet) *
- ☐ Ground Turkey *
- ☐ Trout Fillet*
- ☐ Tuna *
- ☐ Turkey Breast Tenderloin – 3*
- ☐ White Fish *

*amount varies by gender
(see meal plan)*

AVOID GMO FOODS

It is estimated that between 70 and 85 percent of processed foods that we find in our local grocery stores contain GMO ingredients. The FDA does not require labels to inform you of GMOs in your food, so technically there is no way to be sure of the exact percentage that we consume. Some GMO foods include tomatoes, potatoes, squash, golden rice, animal feed, and even farm-raised salmon.

As you can see, grains and corn, among other raw ingredients, are not even close to what they used to be. One chief side effect of these alterations is the inflammation they cause in our bodies, and I see that on a daily basis.

The seven foods listed below are almost always GMO and, therefore, one should choose organic foods, which do not contain GMOs.

1. Corn (88 percent)—popular ingredient in processed food and a staple of animal feed

2. Soy (93 percent)—hydrogenated oils, lecithin, emulsifiers, tocopherol (a vitamin E supplement), and proteins

3. Cottonseed (94 percent)—vegetable oil, margarine or shortening production, fried foods such as potato chips

4. Canola (90 percent)—canola oil is used in cooking, as well as biofuels

5. Sugar beets (90 percent)—sugar beets produce 54% of sugar sold in United States

6. Papaya (75 percent of Hawaiian papaya crop)

7. Alfalfa—no GMO alfalfa on market, but farmers feed it to dairy cows

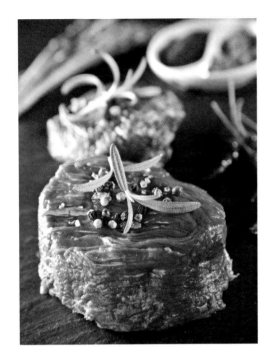

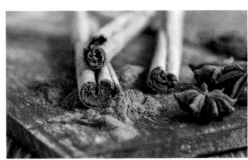

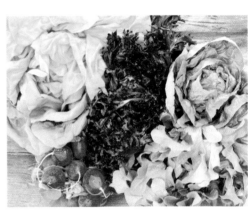

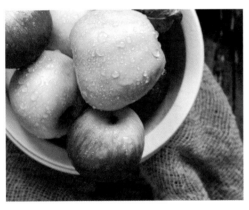

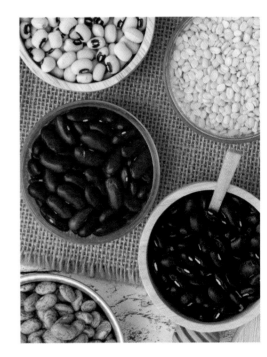

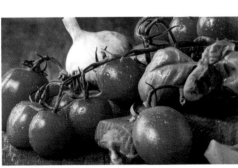

DAY 15

FOUR BEAN SALAD
Yield: 6 servings

The hardest part of this recipe is waiting for the flavors to meld in the refrigerator. You can use dried beans instead of canned, using the recipe from page 95. Parsley may be substituted if you don't have fresh basil. Serve it as a side dish or over mixed salad greens.

⅔ cup apple cider vinegar

⅓ cup extra-virgin oil

3 garlic cloves, peeled and minced

2 teaspoon chopped fresh basil

1 teaspoon dried tarragon

¼ teaspoon black pepper

1 (15-ounce) can light red kidney beans, drained and rinsed

1 (15-ounce) can Northern or white beans, drained and rinsed

1 (15-ounce) can black beans, drained and rinsed

1 (15-ounce) can garbanzo beans, drained and rinsed

1 green bell pepper, seeded and chopped

2 shallots, peeled and minced

1. In a jar with a tight-fitting lid, combine the vinegar, oil, garlic, basil, tarragon, and black pepper. Close and shake to emulsify. Set aside.

2. In a mixing bowl, stir together the kidney beans, white beans, black beans, garbanzo beans, chopped bell pepper pieces, and shallots.

3. Shake the dressing again and pour over the bean mixture. Toss to evenly coat.

4. Cover and refrigerate at least 2 hours.

5. Remove from the refrigerator at least 30 minutes before ready to serve.

6. Toss again and serve alone or over mixed salad greens.

FOOD FACT: BEANS

Storage: Dried beans have one big requirement, which is to be kept dry. They can be stored in their original plastic bag or in a canister on the pantry shelf. Mine usually go into the appropriate sized canning jar so I can easily see the various types I have on hand. Many believe the storage life of dried beans is indefinite, but it is best to use them within one year of purchase for the least amount of soaking time required.

FALL APPLE SOUP
Yield: 4 servings

Although you can enjoy apples all year, there is nothing quite like a trip to a local orchard in the fall. In this dish, Fennel adds a marvelous layer of interest.

2 large Golden Delicious apples, cored, peeled, and chopped
3 carrots, peeled and sliced
2 garlic cloves, peeled and minced
1 small sweet onion, peeled and coarsely chopped
½ cup chopped fennel bulb
2 cups low sodium organic chicken stock (see page 117)
2 cups water
½ cup dry white wine or water
1 bay leaf
¼ teaspoon black pepper
¼ teaspoon dried thyme
¼ teaspoon dried parsley
Plain nonfat yogurt for garnish

1. In a large Dutch oven over medium-high heat, combine the apples, carrots, garlic, chopped onion pieces, fennel, stock, water, wine, bay leaf, pepper, thyme, and parsley.
2. Bring to a boil, then cover and reduce the heat to low.
3. Cook 25 minutes, stirring occasionally.
4. Remove and discard the bay leaf and allow the soup to cool for 10 minutes uncovered.
5. With an immersion blender, puree the soup until smooth.
6. Reheat slightly if necessary.
7. Serve warm with a tablespoon dollop of yogurt on top.

FOOD FACT: FENNEL

Storage: Tightly wrap in plastic, fennel can be refrigerated for five days or longer.

WINTER TOMATOES
Yield: 1 to 2 servings

You probably saw the name of this recipe and wanted to skip right past it. But this is a great way to give juiceless winter tomatoes some taste. Use it as a side, or chop and add to your daily salad.

1 large tomato, cored and sliced
½ teaspoon balsamic vinegar
½ teaspoon dried basil
¼ teaspoon black pepper
⅛ teaspoon garlic salt

1. Place the tomato slices in a single layer on a baking sheet.
2. Drizzle the slices evenly with the vinegar, then sprinkle with the basil, pepper, and salt.
3. Allow to stand at least 15 minutes before serving.

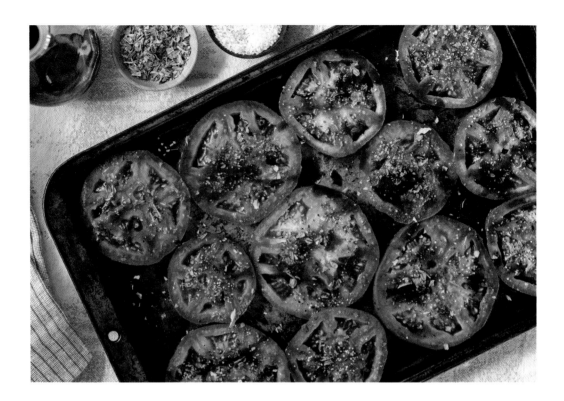

FIFTEEN-MINUTE VEGETABLE CHILI
Yield: 4 servings

Unlike chili recipes that require an entire day in the slow cooker, this one is almost instant. You can use dried beans instead of canned, cooked per the recipe found on page 95. And you will not miss the meat!

2 garlic cloves, peeled and minced

2 large carrots, peeled and
    coarsely grated

2½ cups tomato puree

2½ cups low sodium vegetable
    stock or water (see page 96)

3 tablespoons tomato paste

2 (15-ounce) cans black beans,
    drained and rinsed

1 (15-ounce) can light red kidney beans

1 jalapeno pepper, seeded and minced

1 teaspoon chili powder

½ teaspoon onion salt

¼ teaspoon black pepper

1. Place the garlic, carrots, tomato puree, stock, tomato paste, black beans, kidney beans, jalapeno, chili powder, salt, and pepper in a large saucepan or Dutch oven.

2. Place over high heat and cook for 15 minutes. Serve warm.

Fruited Beef & Barley Salad
Yield: 4 servings

This is a recipe you can pull out anytime to impress guests or for a special occasion. The charred bell peppers add a nice color pop and your kitchen will smell marvelous as it all roasts.

1 pound lean beef sirloin tri-tip roast
1½ teaspoons paprika, divided
1 large red bell pepper, seeded and cut in cubes
1 large orange bell pepper, seeded and cut in cubes
1 cup quick-cooking barley
3 limes, juiced
1 teaspoon extra-virgin oil
¼ teaspoon black pepper
¼ teaspoon dried parsley
2 mangos, peeled and cubed
4 green onions, chopped
¼ cup chopped fresh cilantro
Mixed salad greens

1. Preheat the oven to 425 degrees.
2. Place the roast on a lightly greased roasting pan and rub 1 teaspoon of the paprika over the top surface.
3. Insert a meat thermometer and roast for 40 minutes.
4. Coat a baking sheet with cooking spray and add the bell peppers.
5. Place in the oven with the roast during the last 25 minutes of cooking.
6. The meat thermometer should read 135 degrees for medium rare or 150 degrees for medium.
7. Remove the thermometer and tent with foil. Let stand 15 minutes.
8. Meanwhile, prepare the barley according to the package directions and set aside.
9. Place the lime juice, oil, black pepper, and parsley in a jar with a tight fitting lid. Cover and shake to emulsify then set aside.
10. Cut the roast in bit-sized pieces and add to a large bowl along with the bell peppers, mangos, green onions, and cilantro.
11. Toss with the dressing and transfer on top of mixed salad greens. Serve immediately.

Fuji Apple Crumble
Yield: 2 servings

With just a couple of apples, you can have a special treat that mimics a traditional crisp or crumble recipe. You can also make this recipe with any leftover stewed apples. You may substitute pears for the apples, if desired.

2 Fuji apples, peeled, cored and cut in slices
¼ cup apple juice or cider
¼ cup golden raisins or dried cranberries

1 tablespoon unsalted, grass-fed butter

¼ cup rolled oats

1 heaping tablespoon sunflower seeds

1-2 teaspoon organic stevia

2 tablespoons plain Greek yogurt

1. Place the apples and juice in a small saucepan over medium-high heat.
2. Bring to a boil and reduce the heat to low.
3. Simmer for 3 minutes and add the raisins.
4. Cover and remove from the heat.
5. In a small frying pan, melt the butter over medium-high heat.
6. Add the oats and seeds and cook, stirring constantly for 2 minutes.
7. Add the stevia and remove from the heat.
8. Divide the apple mixture among serving bowls and top evenly with the oat mixture.
9. Garnish each with a tablespoon of yogurt and serve warm.

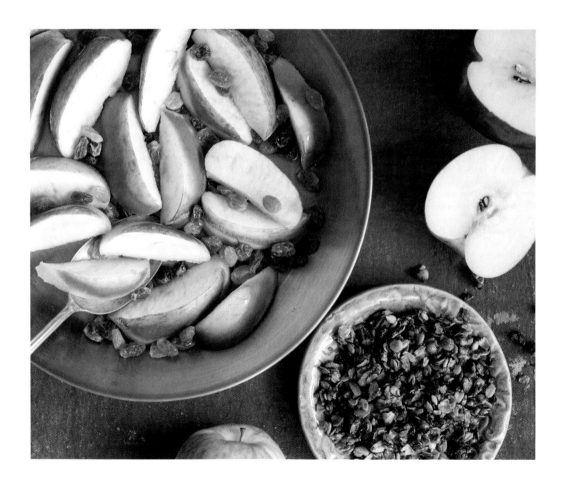

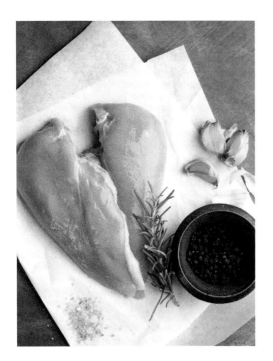

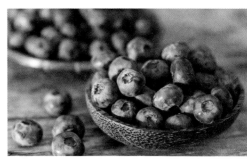

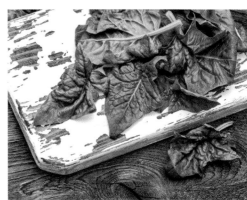

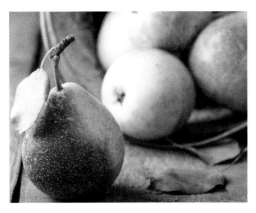

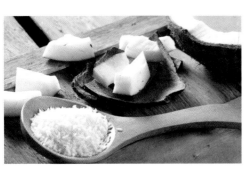

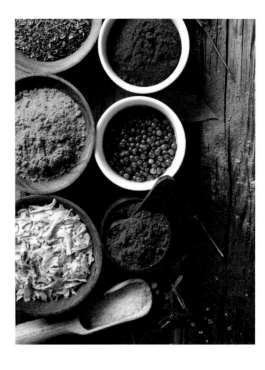

DAY 16

PEAR-SPIKED CARROT SOUP
Yield: 4 servings

This is a soup for any type of weather because it is just as exceptional served at room temperature as it is hot or cold. It is just right for fall when pears are in season.

2 tablespoons extra-virgin oil

1 sweet onion, peeled and sliced

2 garlic cloves, peeled and minced

1 tablespoon curry powder

8 cups low sodium, organic vegetable or chicken stock (see page 96 or 117)

5 carrots, peeled and coarsely chopped

2 ripe pears, cored, peeled, and sliced

1 tablespoon firmly packed light brown sugar

2 tablespoons lemon juice

½ teaspoon salt

¼ teaspoon black pepper

Chopped fresh parsley for garnish

1. Place the oil in a Dutch oven over medium heat.
2. When hot, add the sliced onion pieces and cook for 3 minutes, stirring frequently.
3. Add the garlic and curry powder. Cook 1 minute longer, stirring constantly.
4. Add the stock, carrots, pears, and sugar.
5. Bring to a boil and reduce the heat to low.
6. Simmer uncovered for 20 minutes.
7. Remove from the heat and puree with an immersion blender.
8. Stir in the lemon juice, salt, and pepper.
9. Garnish with the parsley and serve warm.

FOOD FACT: CHICKEN

If you purchase chicken with the skin still attached, don't worry! The skin can be left on during cooking to naturally moisturize the cut. Then when you are ready to serve, it can easily be removed. If you prefer to remove it before cooking, pull to loosen it from the meat and cut away with poultry shears.

ROSEMARY CHICKEN
Yield: 2 servings

Variety is imperative for keeping things interesting on the dinner plate and keeping you on track with your meal plan. The herb garden is a great place to mix things up a bit while using a tried and true recipe that you can learn to do without thinking. Start with the rosemary suggested, then venture into other herbs and herb combinations.

2 boneless, skinless chicken breasts

1 lemon, cut in half

1 large clove garlic, peeled and minced

1 tablespoon chopped fresh rosemary,
divided

½ teaspoon onion salt

¼ teaspoon black pepper

1. Preheat the oven to 375 degrees.
2. Place the chicken on a greased baking sheet and spray the top of each piece with cooking spray.
3. Zest half of the lemon and squeeze the juice over the chicken.
4. Cut the remaining lemon half into wedges and set aside.
5. Sprinkle the zest, half of the rosemary, salt and pepper evenly on both sides of the chicken.
6. Bake for 20 minutes.
7. Set the broiler on high and lightly brown on the top.
8. Sprinkle with the remaining rosemary and serve warm with the lemon wedges.

FOOD FACT: PEPPERS

Freeze: Raw peppers are one of only two vegetables that do not have to be blanched before freezing. The other is onions. So chop any excess and store in small amounts in your freezer. Use within one year.

CHUNKY REFRIED BEAN DIP
Yield: 2 cups

Although pinto beans are traditionally used in refried beans, any leftover cooked beans will do just fine. Try red beans, black beans, kidney beans, white beans, or even a combination!

2 teaspoon extra-virgin oil

1 medium sweet onion, peeled and
chopped

4 garlic cloves, peeled and minced

1 jalapeno pepper, seeded and
minced

1 small red bell pepper, seeded
and finely chopped

½ teaspoon ground cumin

½ teaspoon chili powder

¼ teaspoon ground coriander

¼ teaspoon black pepper

¼ teaspoon paprika

2 cups cooked pinto beans, room
temperature and mashed

1 tablespoon lemon juice

1 tablespoon water

1. Place the oil in a medium saucepan over medium-high heat.
2. When hot, add the chopped onion pieces, garlic, and jalapeno pepper.
3. Cook 2 minutes, stirring frequently.
4. Add the chopped red bell pepper pieces, cumin, chili powder, coriander, black pepper, and paprika. Cook another 2 minutes.

5. Reduce the heat to low and stir in the beans, lemon juice, and water. Cook, stirring constantly until the mixture is thoroughly combined and warm.

6. Serve immediately or cool to room temperature and serve.

SPINACH CHIVE MUFFINS
Yield: about 16 muffins

These muffins are loaded with spinach and have a hint of delicate chives. You can pair them with ordinary tomato soup or grab one for a savory breakfast treat.

3 cups gluten-free all-purpose flour
1 tablespoon baking powder
1 tablespoon dried chives
1¼ teaspoons garlic salt
½ teaspoon white pepper
½ teaspoon baking soda
¾ cup almond, coconut, or
    nonfat milk
¾ cup plain nonfat yogurt
½ cup extra-virgin oil
1 (10-ounce) package frozen
    chopped spinach, thawed and
    squeezed dry

1. Preheat the oven to 400 degrees.
2. Line 16 muffin cups with paper liners and set aside.

3. In a mixing bowl, stir together the flour, baking powder, chives, salt, pepper, and baking soda.

4. In a separate bowl, whisk together the milk, yogurt, oil, and spinach.

5. Add to the flour mixture and stir just until blended.

6. Divide the batter evenly among the muffin cups.

7. Bake for 18-20 minutes or until a cake tester inserted in the center comes out clean.

8. Let cool in the pan on a wire rack for 3 minutes.

9. Remove from the pan and cool completely on the rack.

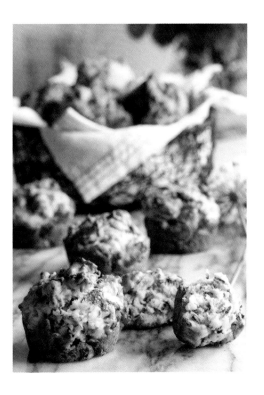

PAN-BLACKENED SNAPPER
Yield: 2 servings

The flavor punch you get from rubbing fish with seasoning, then placing it in a red-hot cast iron skillet is unmatched. It sears the fish, giving it a nice crisp "crust" without the fat of deep frying. The key to success is letting the skillet thoroughly preheat on the stove. Make sure your exhaust fan is on high.

> 2 snapper fillets
> 1 tablespoon lemon juice
> ½ teaspoon dried thyme
> ½ teaspoon onion or garlic salt
> ½ teaspoon paprika
> ¼ teaspoon cayenne
> ¼ teaspoon black pepper
> 2 teaspoons extra-virgin oil
> Lemon wedges for serving

1. Place a large cast iron skillet over medium-high heat.

2. Place the snapper fillets on a greased baking sheet and brush with the lemon juice.
3. In a small bowl, combine the thyme, salt, cayenne, pepper, and paprika.
4. Rub evenly on both sides of the fish fillets, using ½ teaspoon of the mixture on each side.
5. Add the oil to the skillet and after 30 seconds, add the fish.
6. Cook 3 minutes on each side or until the fish flakes easily with a fork. Serve immediately.

BLUEBERRY OAT SQUARES
Yield: 12 squares

Anytime you can incorporate fruit into a dessert treat is a plus. These require some resting time in the refrigerator, but they are worth the wait!

> 1 cup rolled oats
> ½ cup natural peanut butter
> ½ cup unsweetened shredded coconut
> ⅓ cup coconut oil, melted
> ⅓ cup pure maple syrup
> 1 teaspoon pure vanilla extract
> 1 cup fresh blueberries

1. Place parchment paper onto the bottom and up the sides of an 8-inch square baking pan and set aside.

2. In a mixing bowl, stir together the oats, peanut butter, coconut, oil, syrup, and extract.

3. Transfer to the prepared baking pan and press in the bottom.

4. Top with the blueberries, gently pressing into the crust.

5. Cover and refrigerate for 2 hours before slicing into squares and serving.

FOOD FACT: PEANUTS

Peanut butter was invented in 1890 by a St. Louis physician who was seeking a nutritious, easily digested, high protein food for some of his elderly patients with poor teeth that couldn't chew meat.

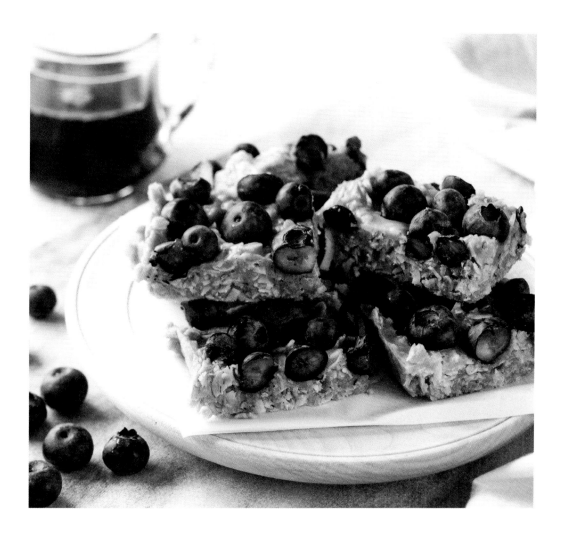

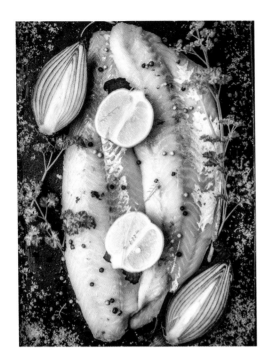
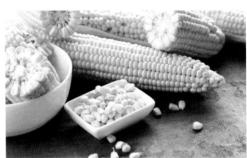
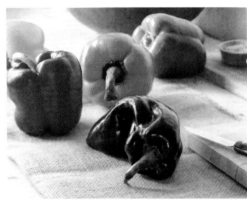
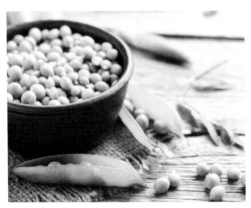
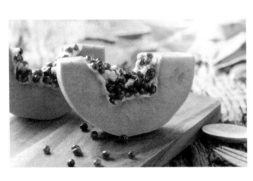
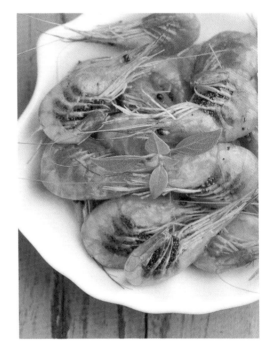

DAY 17

SUMMER EDAMAME SALAD
Yield: 4 servings

This side dish salad has all the ingredients of a summer garden rolled into one delightful dish. It's quickly prepared in one dish, going from pantry to plate in less than 10 minutes.

2 cups shelled edamame

1½ cups whole kernel corn

1 (15-ounce) can black beans, drained and rinsed

3 Roma tomatoes, chopped

1 large shallot, peeled and chopped

¼ cup chopped fresh cilantro

3 tablespoons lime juice

1 tablespoon extra-virgin oil

½ teaspoon cayenne

¼ teaspoon black pepper

Mixed salad greens

1. In a large bowl, toss together the edamame, corn, beans, tomatoes, chopped shallot pieces, and cilantro.
2. Drizzle with the lime juice and oil and sprinkle with the cayenne and black pepper.
3. Toss to evenly coat. Serve at room temperature over mixed salad greens or cover and refrigerate for later use.

FOOD FACT: CORN

Storage: Fresh corn should be used as quickly as possible, but until you can get it prepared, keep it refrigerated in a plastic bag.

SOUTHWESTERN SALAD
Yield: 2 servings

The work horse of the bean family has to be versatile black beans. Here they serve as the vehicle for showcasing sweet corn and equally sweet red bell peppers. Heat it up with more chopped jalapeno peppers if you wish.

3 large ears sweet corn, kernels cut from the cob

2 green onions, chopped

1 large red bell pepper, seeded and chopped

1 jalapeno pepper, seeded and finely chopped

1 (15.5-ounce) can black beans, drained and rinsed

3 tablespoons chopped fresh cilantro, divided

2 tablespoons lime juice
2 tablespoons extra-virgin oil
½ teaspoon onion salt
¼ teaspoon black pepper
Mixed salad greens

1. In a mixing bowl, combine the corn, onions, chopped bell pepper and jalapeno pepper pieces,beans, 2 tablespoons of the cilantro, lime juice, oil, salt, and pepper.
2. Let stand at room temperature 20 minutes.
3. Serve over mixed salad greens with a garnish of the remaining cilantro.

Fresh Fish Tacos with Lime
Yield: 2 servings

Lime juice enhances nearly any type of fish, and I love the extra zing it gets from fresh cilantro. Here, it's paired with warm gluten-free tortillas, but it is just as exceptional served on a bed of fresh salad greens.

2 halibut, snapper, or tilapia fillets
1 tablespoon + 2 teaspoons lime juice
1 tablespoon extra-virgin oil
½ teaspoon salt, divided
¼ teaspoon black pepper
⅓ cup plain Greek yogurt
2 tablespoons chopped fresh cilantro
4 gluten-free tortillas
Chopped lettuce

1. Preheat the oven to 425 degrees and lightly spray a baking sheet with cooking spray.
2. Add the fillets and sprinkle evenly with 1 tablespoon of the juice, the oil, ¼ teaspoon of the salt, and the pepper.
3. Bake for 10 minutes or until the fish flakes easily with a fork.
4. Meanwhile, whisk together the yogurt, cilantro, the remaining lime juice, and salt in a small bowl. Set aside.
5. Wrap the tortillas in a slightly damp dish towel and place in a covered oven-safe dish.
6. When the fish is done, turn off the oven and remove, but add the tortilla dish to warm.
7. Flake the fish and add along with the chopped lettuce to the warm tortillas.
8. Drizzle with the cilantro dressing and serve warm.

Option #2:
Use the same ingredients as if making tacos with fish, except use 2 boneless, skinless chicken breasts instead of fish fillets.

1. Follow same steps as if making fish tacos.
2. Bake chicken for 20 minutes, or until the chicken is done.
3. Cut cooked chicken into thin slices.

FOOD FACT: WATERMELONS

Selecting Pieces: There is nothing wrong with purchasing watermelon that has already been cut, but you'll pay more than if you bought a whole melon. That goes back to the standard food rule: "The more it's cut, the more it costs!" For small families, however, cut melons are a great solution for eliminating waste. Look for a bright flesh that appears moist. If it has seeds, they should be brown or black. Seeds that are white are immature, which is only desirable in "seedless" melons.

FRUIT SALSA
Yield: about 2-½ cups

Let your imagination soar with this recipe. You can use all sorts of fresh fruits to lend a unique flavor to this salsa. In addition to the papaya, try cantaloupe, watermelon, and even mango! It is delicious on toasted whole wheat or gluten-free bread or with baked tortilla chips (see page 125).

- 1 papaya, peeled, seeded, and chopped
- 4 Roma tomatoes, chopped
- 2 garlic cloves, peeled and minced
- ½ small red onion, peeled and chopped
- ¼ cup chopped fresh cilantro
- ¼ cup chopped fresh parsley
- 1 tablespoon lime juice
- ¼ teaspoon black pepper

1. In a medium bowl, combine the papaya, tomatoes, garlic, chopped onion pieces, cilantro, parsley, lime juice, and pepper.
2. Cover and let stand for 30 minutes or refrigerate for later use.

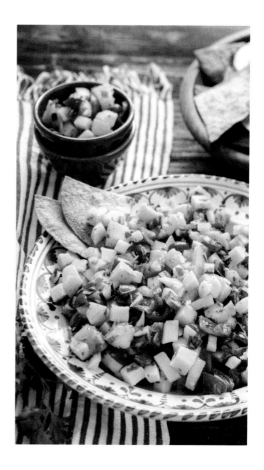

ZESTY GARLIC SHRIMP STEW
Yield: 4 servings

This recipe calls for a whole head of garlic, but because it's roasted, you have a mellow garlic flavor rather than an overpowering one. You can easily substitute another protein for the shrimp, such as lump crab meat or leftover chicken, turkey, or pork.

1 garlic bulb
1 tablespoon extra-virgin oil
3 celery stalks, trimmed and chopped
1 large red bell pepper, seeded and
    chopped
1 large orange bell pepper, seeded and
    chopped
1 small leek, trimmed and thinly sliced
1 jalapeno pepper, seeded and minced
2½ cups tomatoes, peeled and chopped
    (seeded if desired)
3 cups low sodium, organic chicken
    stock (see page 117)
½ teaspoon dried oregano
½ teaspoon paprika
½ teaspoon cayenne
½ teaspoon black pepper
1 cup whole kernel corn
1 pound small shrimp, peeled and
    deveined
Chopped fresh parsley for garnish

1. Preheat the oven to 350 degrees.
2. Trim the top half-inch of the garlic bulb and place on a piece of parchment paper.
3. Moisten it with a tablespoon or two of water.
4. Wrap up the parchment paper and tightly seal, stapling paper if necessary.
5. Place on a baking sheet and bake for 45 minutes.
6. Remove and set aside to cool.
7. Place the oil in a Dutch oven over medium-high heat.
8. When hot, add the garlic, celery, bell peppers, leeks, and jalapenos.
9. Cook for 10 minutes, stirring frequently.
10. Add the tomatoes, stock, oregano, paprika, cayenne, and black pepper.
11. Bring to a simmer and add the corn and shrimp. Cook for 3 minutes.
12. Serve warm with a garnish of fresh parsley.

VEGETABLE STUFFED PEPPERS
Yield: 2 servings

This recipe takes vegetables you might serve separately and bakes them in a garden-fresh bell pepper. Use it as a guide for stuffing peppers with anything you have lingering in the fridge that needs to be used up.

2 large green bell peppers
1 Roma tomato, diced
1 small shallot, peeled and minced
1 garlic clove, peeled and minced
¾ cup whole kernel corn
¾ cup cooked beans (pinto, black,
    garbanzo, lima, kidney, or white)

2 tablespoons shredded cheese
(Cheddar, Swiss or Monterey Jack)

1 tablespoon pine nuts

1 teaspoon extra-virgin oil

1 teaspoon chopped fresh parsley

¼ teaspoon black pepper

¼ teaspoon cayenne

1. Bring a large saucepan of water to a boil over high heat.
2. Cut peppers in half horizontally, leaving tops intact. Remove seeds and inner ribs.
3. Immerse the peppers in the boiling water and cook for 5 minutes.
4. Meanwhile, preheat the oven to 375 degrees.
5. In a medium bowl, combine the diced tomato pieces, shallot, garlic, corn, beans, cheese, pine nuts, oil, parsley, black pepper, and cayenne. Stir well and set aside.
6. With tongs, remove the peppers from the water and drain upside down on paper towels.
7. Fill the peppers by evenly dividing the vegetable mixture between each.
8. Place in a baking dish and add ¼ cup of water in the bottom of the dish.
9. Bake for 20 minutes.
10. Let rest 5 minutes before serving warm.

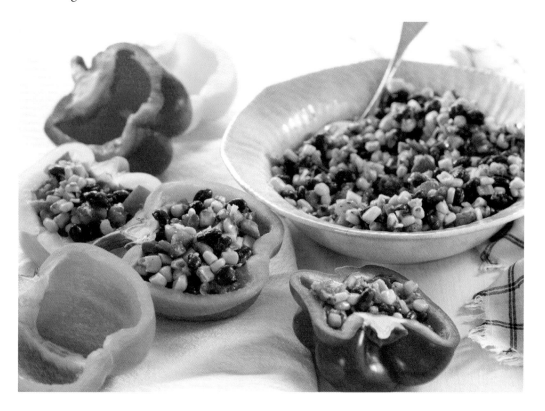

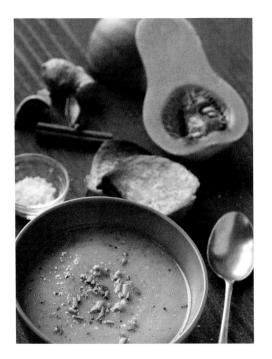

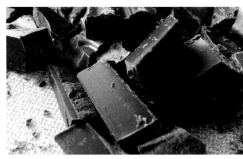

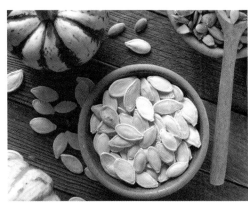

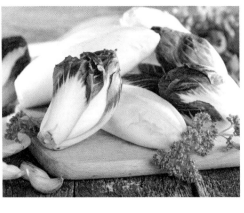

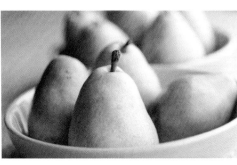

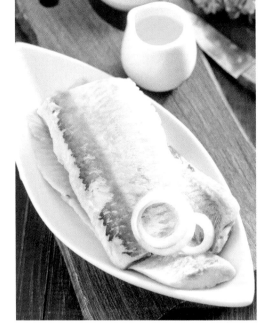

DAY 18

DARK CHOCOLATE STRAWBERRIES
Yield: 3 servings

This is not a dish to make in the spring when local strawberries are widely available. Instead, use it to enhance out-of-season fruit that doesn't have the natural sweetness of those grown down the street.

    4 ounces dark chocolate (65-75 percent cacao), chopped
    2 teaspoons avocado or coconut oil
    12 strawberries with stems attached

1. Place a wire rack over a baking sheet that has been lined with waxed paper and set aside.
2. Place the chocolate and shortening in a small bowl and microwave on medium power for 15 seconds. Stir and if additional time is needed, only do so in 5 second intervals, stirring after each.
3. Holding each strawberry by the stem and close to the cap, dip halfway in the melted chocolate.
4. Place on the prepared rack, tilting the berry so it rests on the shoulder or cap.
5. Allow to stand for 15 minutes to harden before serving.

FOOD FACT: DARK CHOCOLATE

Eating dark chocolate with stevia instead of sugar a couple times a day boosts dopamine levels, helps turn off food cravings, and improves blood flow to the brain.

SPICED WINTER SQUASH SOUP
Yield: 6 servings

Even though you can use any winter squash variety to make this soup, reach for butternut. The texture is almost creamy.

    2 tablespoons extra-virgin oil
    1 sweet onion, peeled and chopped
    3 garlic cloves, peeled and minced
    1 tablespoon gluten-free all-purpose flour
    8 cups low sodium vegetable or chicken stock (see page 96 or 117)
    1 butternut squash, peeled, seeded and cubed
    4 cups coarsely chopped Chinese cabbage
    ½ fennel bulb, coarsely chopped
    1¼ teaspoons ground cumin
    1 teaspoon mustard seeds

½ teaspoon crushed red pepper

½ teaspoon fennel seeds

½ teaspoon salt

¼ teaspoon black pepper

1. Place the oil in a Dutch oven over medium heat.
2. When hot, add the chopped onion pieces and cook, stirring frequently for 3 minutes.
3. Add the garlic and cook 1 minute, stirring constantly.
4. Sprinkle with the flour and cook 1 minute, stirring constantly.
5. Gradually whisk in the stock and bring to a boil.
6. Add the squash, cabbage, and fennel and reduce the heat to low. Simmer uncovered for 20 minutes.
7. Stir in the cumin, mustard seeds, crushed red pepper, fennel seeds, salt, and black pepper.
8. Cook 12 minutes longer and remove from the heat.
9. With an immersion blender, puree the soup until smooth or the desired texture is achieved. Serve warm.

Pear & Pumpkin Seed Salad
Yield: 2 servings

The classic combination of pears and pumpkin seeds gets a unique twist with endive. It feels extravagant . . . like you are getting a treat!

1 ripe pear, cored, peeled, and thinly sliced

Juice of ½ lemon

2 heads endive, trimmed and thinly sliced in rounds

¼ cup pumpkin seeds

2 tablespoons crumbled blue cheese

1 tablespoon extra-virgin oil

¼ teaspoon salt

¼ teaspoon black pepper

1. Place the pear slices in a shallow bowl and add the lemon juice, tossing to evenly coat. Set aside.
2. Divide the endive between 2 plates.
3. Top each with half of the pumpkin seeds and cheese, then with the pear slices.
4. Mix any lemon juice remaining in the bowl with the oil, salt and pepper.
5. Drizzle over the salads and serve immediately.

FOOD FACT: PUMPKIN

The word "pumpkin" comes from the medieval European term for squash, "pompion." It progressed to popon, pompon, pumpion and eventually pumpkin. The seeds are sometimes marketed under the Mexican term "pepitas". Pumpkin seeds can be purchased with or without the hulls.

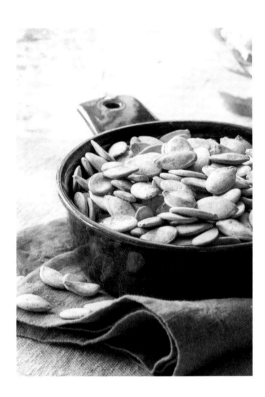

1. Preheat the oven to 300 degrees and line a baking sheet with parchment paper. Set aside.
2. In a mixing bowl, combine the seeds, oil, and sweet or savory seasonings.
3. Spread in a single layer in the baking sheet.
4. Bake for 40 minutes or until golden brown, stirring halfway through.
5. Cool and store at room temperature in an airtight container.

HERBED BROILED MUSHROOMS
Yield: 2 servings

Portabella are the culinary giants of all mushrooms. They have an unbeatable flavor and command attention on the plate. Here they are quickly broiled with an herb-enhanced oil that can be a side dish, a salad topping, or a sandwich star.

    4 portabella mushrooms
    2 tablespoons extra-virgin oil
    1 small garlic clove, peeled and
        minced
    ¼ teaspoon dried basil
    ⅛ teaspoon black pepper
    ⅛ teaspoon salt
    1 teaspoon fresh snipped chives
    1 teaspoon chopped fresh parsley

1. Preheat the broiler to high and line a baking sheet with aluminum foil.

ROASTED PUMPKIN SEEDS
Yield: 2 cups

You'll need a little more time to roast raw pumpkin seeds than you will roasting traditional nuts, but it's an easy thing to do while you are doing other kitchen chores. Here are flavor options for sweet and savory.

    2 cups raw whole pumpkin seeds
    2 teaspoons extra-virgin oil
    1 teaspoon ground cinnamon
        (for sweet) or chili powder
        (for savory)
    ½ teaspoon brown sugar (for sweet)
        or garlic powder (for savory)

2. Place the mushrooms with the stem side up on the baking sheet.
3. In a small bowl, whisk together the oil, garlic, basil, pepper, and salt.
4. Brush over the upturned sides of the mushrooms.
5. Broil for 4 minutes.
6. Remove from the oven and let rest for 1 minute.
7. Sprinkle with the chives and parsley and serve warm.

Pan-Roasted Fish with Orange Glaze
Yield: 2 servings

If you have a cast-iron skillet, pull it out now. Along with stove-top heat, it gives any fish you select a nice crust. Give this recipe your full attention because the fish will be done in a flash.

> 2 tablespoons extra-virgin oil
> 2 (no more than 1-inch thick) fish fillets
> ½ teaspoon onion salt
> ¼ teaspoon black pepper
> 2 tablespoons low calorie orange marmalade
> 1 tablespoon chopped fresh parsley

1. Place the oil in a large cast-iron skillet over high heat.

2. Season the fillets with the salt and pepper.
3. When hot, add the fillets to the pan, holding down for around 15 seconds with a spatula to prevent curling.
4. Immediately reduce the heat to medium and allow the fillets to cook for 2 minutes or until evenly browned. Carefully flip and cook 1 minute.
5. Add the marmalade and cook another minute.
6. Top with the fresh parsley and serve immediately.

FOOD FACT: FISH

Tilapia: Tilapia is sometimes called St. Peter's fish or Hawaiian sunfish. It has a remarkably sweet flavor, and the flesh is white and occasionally slightly pink.

Haddock: Haddock is a close relative of cod and is a saltwater fish that ranges from 2-6 pounds.

Mackerel: Mackerel is sometimes sold smoked or salted. If you purchase salted, it should be soaked in cold water overnight to remove the excess salt before using.

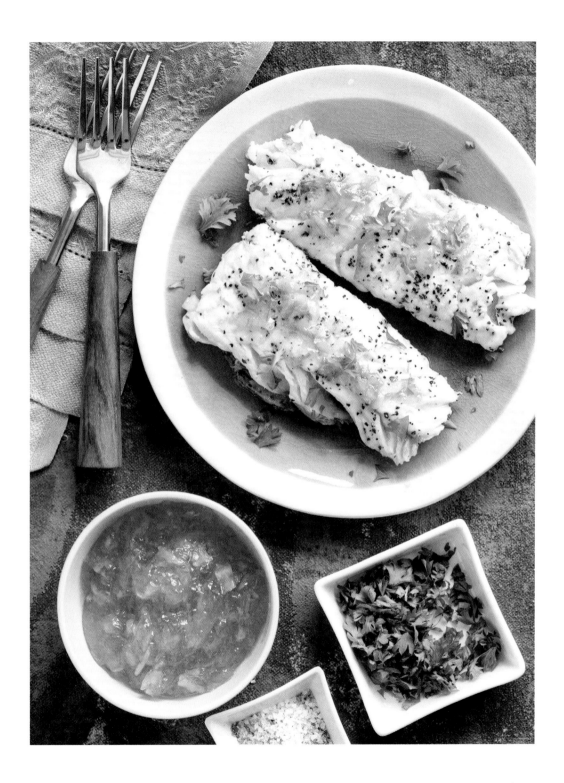

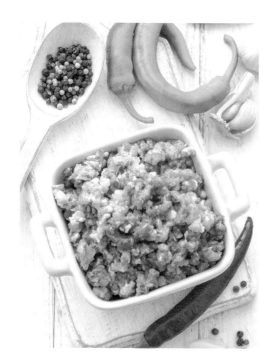

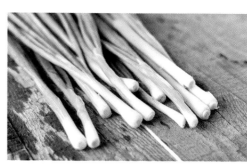

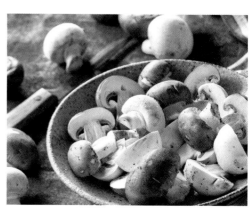

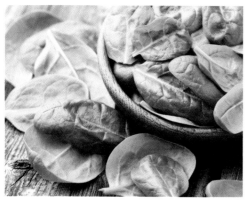

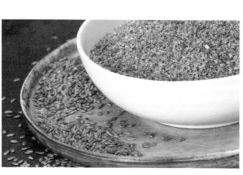

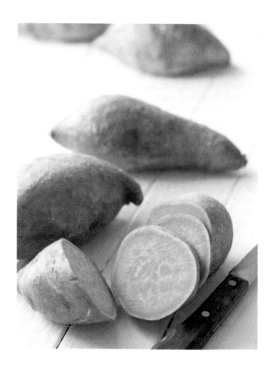

DAY 19

FRUIT & FLAX MUFFINS
Yield: about 12 muffins

This is a do-ahead muffin recipe that is worth the planning. Use dried sour cherries or cranberries. There is something about the tart punch that really wakes up the taste buds in the morning.

 1¾ cups almond, coconut, or nonfat milk
 1 tablespoon apple cider vinegar
 1 cup chopped dried fruit
 1 cup old-fashioned rolled oats
 ½ cup bran cereal
 ½ cup extra-virgin oil
 ⅓ cup sugar
 ¼ ground flaxseeds or chia seeds
 ¼ teaspoon salt
 ½ cup boiling water
 1½ cups gluten-free all-purpose flour
 1¼ teaspoons baking soda
 1 teaspoon ground cinnamon

1. In a 2-cup measuring cup, stir together the milk and vinegar. Let stand for 5 minutes while you measure the remaining ingredients.
2. In a mixing bowl, stir together the fruit, oats, cereal, oil, sugar, flaxseeds, and salt.
3. Add the boiling water and mix well.
4. Stir in the milk mixture and set aside to cool for 30 minutes.
5. Preheat the oven to 375 degrees.
6. Line 12 muffin cups with paper liners and set aside.
7. In a medium bowl, stir together the flour, baking soda, and cinnamon. Add to the cooled fruit mixture and stir just until blended.
8. Evenly divide the batter among the muffin cups, filling no more than two-thirds full.
9. Bake 18-21 minutes or until a cake tester inserted in the center comes out clean. The tops will be golden brown.
10. Cool in the pan 3 minutes, then transfer to a wire rack to cool completely.

FOOD FACT: FLAXSEEDS

Storage: The omega-3 fatty acids in flaxseeds shorten the shelf life if not stored correctly. These fatty acids are a boost for our health, but can turn rancid if kept at room temperature. Place in a freezer container and it will keep there for up to eight months. If you prefer refrigerator storage, it will keep between four and five months.

GARLIC & GINGER GREEN BEANS
Yield: 2 to 3 servings

Forget about cooking green beans for long periods of time on the stove. These are quickly boiled in stock, then added to sautéed shallot pieces, garlic, and ginger to create a flavorful enhancement for a meat dish.

3 cups low sodium organic vegetable or chicken stock (see page 96 or 117)
1 pound fresh green beans, trimmed
1 tablespoon extra-virgin oil
1 shallot, peeled and chopped
2 garlic cloves, peeled and minced
1 tablespoon fresh minced ginger
¼ teaspoon salt
¼ teaspoon black pepper

1. Place the stock in a large saucepan over high heat and bring to a boil.
2. Add the green beans and cook for 5 to 6 minutes. Drain and set aside.
3. Place the oil in the same saucepan over medium-high heat.
4. When hot, add the chopped shallot pieces. Cook 3 minutes, stirring frequently.
5. Add the garlic and ginger and cook 1 minute longer.
6. Return the green beans to the saucepan along with the salt and pepper.
7. Remove from the heat and cover. Let stand 2 minutes before serving warm.

FOOD FACT: SPINACH

Spinach is one of the foods known to lower blood sugar, lower triglycerides, prevent cancer, relieve ADHD and Autism, and decrease anxiety.

ROASTED SWEET POTATO SALAD WITH LIME PEPPER DRESSING
Yield: 2 servings

Instead of boiling sweet potatoes, this recipe calls for roasting them in the oven along with a bell pepper and cubed onion. Then the hearty trio is crunched up with celery and a large apple. The dressing is a nice alternative to ordinary oil and vinegar.

1 large sweet potato, peeled and cubed
1 large red bell pepper
¼ sweet onion, peeled and cubed
1 large Granny Smith or Fuji apple
1 small celery stalk, chopped
2 tablespoons chopped fresh cilantro
1 chipotle pepper in adobo
3 tablespoons lime juice
3 tablespoons extra-virgin oil
1 garlic clove, peeled
½ teaspoon stevia
¼ teaspoon black pepper
Baby spinach leaves

1. Preheat the oven to 375 degrees.
2. Place the cubed sweet potato and onion pieces and whole bell pepper on a greased baking sheet in a single layer. Spray the tops lightly with cooking spray.
3. Roast for 25 minutes.
4. Remove from the oven and place the bell pepper in a zip top bag to steam.
5. Allow the sweet potato and onion cubes to cool on the pan.
6. Meanwhile, core and cube the apple and add to a mixing bowl along with the celery and cilantro.
7. Place the chipotle, lime juice, oil, garlic, nectar, and pepper in the bowl of a food processor. Process until smooth.

8. Remove the pepper from the bag. Core, seed, and slice the pepper.
9. Add the bell pepper slices along with the sweet potato and onion cubes to the mixing bowl and toss well to coat.
10. Arrange over baby spinach leaves and drizzle with the dressing. Serve immediately.

TONGAL TUNA SALAD WRAPS
Yield: 2 servings

Using Greek yogurt instead of mayonnaise changes the taste completely—for the better! It gets a tang that is underlined by the lemon juice. The peppery arugula pairs nicely with the sweet red grapes.

2 tablespoons plain nonfat Greek yogurt
1 teaspoon lemon juice
1 (6-ounce) can tongal tuna packed in water, drained
½ cup halved seedless red grapes
1 small celery stalk, chopped
¼ cup chopped walnuts
1 small shallot, peeled and chopped
2 (10-inch) gluten-free, whole wheat, or organic corn tortillas
2 cups arugula

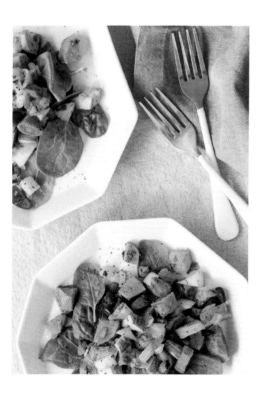

1. In a mixing bowl, whisk together the yogurt and lemon juice.
2. Stir in the tuna, grapes, celery, walnuts, and chopped shallot pieces, mixing well.

3. Place the tortillas on a cutting board and divide the tuna mixture evenly on top.
4. Add the arugula and roll tightly. Secure with toothpicks if necessary and serve.

KICKED-UP TURKEY SOUP
Yield: 4 servings

This has all the elements of a fiesta without the carbs from chips or tortillas. The preparation for this soup is fast and if you don't have fresh tomatoes, you can substitute a can of diced tomatoes with no salt added.

1 tablespoon extra-virgin oil
1 sweet onion, peeled and chopped
1 jalapeno pepper, seeded and minced
1 garlic clove, peeled and minced
1 zucchini, chopped
1½ teaspoons ground cumin
1 teaspoon chili powder
½ teaspoon black pepper
1 pound lean ground turkey
4 cups low sodium chicken stock
(see page 117)
1 cup peeled, diced tomatoes
1 (15-ounce) can black beans, drained and rinsed
1 cup whole kernel corn
½ cup chopped fresh cilantro

1. Place the oil in a Dutch oven over medium-high heat.

2. Add the chopped onion pieces, jalapeno, and garlic. Cook for 5 minutes, stirring frequently.
3. Add the zucchini, cumin, chili powder, and black pepper. Cook for 8 minutes, stirring frequently.
4. Add the ground turkey and cook for 5 minutes, breaking apart with the spoon as it cooks.
5. Stir in the stock, tomatoes, beans, and corn and bring to a boil. Reduce the heat to low and simmer 20 minutes.
6. Remove from the heat and add the cilantro. Serve warm.

FOOD FACT: MUSHROOMS

Selection: No matter which variety you select, firm, fresh-looking mushrooms are best. They should almost appear to be a little moist.

MUSHROOM CAVIAR
Yield: 1½ cups

This snack feels as extravagant as the name leads you to think it is. It is certainly worthy of serving to company and it will make any day feel like a special occasion. Serve it with celery sticks, toasted gluten-free pita bread, or baked tortilla chips (see page 125).

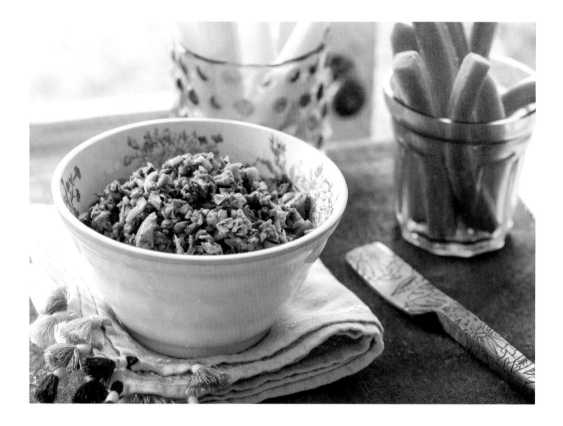

1 tablespoon extra-virgin oil

1 (8-ounce) package sliced
    mushrooms

4 green onions, trimmed and sliced
    (reserve 2 teaspoons green parts
    for garnish)

4 garlic cloves, peeled and minced

½ teaspoon chopped fresh thyme

4 teaspoons balsamic vinegar

2 teaspoon lemon juice

¼ teaspoon black pepper

1. Place the oil in a large skillet over
    medium-high heat.

2. When hot, add the mushrooms, onions,
    and garlic. Cook 7 minutes and remove
    from the heat.

3. Stir in the thyme and allow to cool for
    15 minutes.

4. Transfer to the food processor and
    pulse until coarsely chopped. Do not
    over process.

5. Return to the skillet and add the
    vinegar, lemon juice, and pepper.

6. Place over medium-high heat and
    cook for 10 minutes longer or until
    the liquid has nearly evaporated.

7. Serve warm or at room temperature.

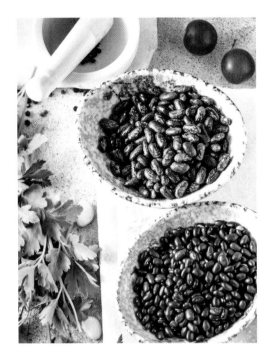
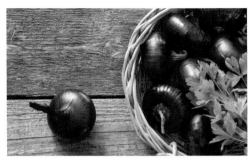
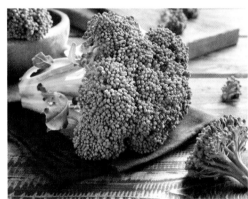
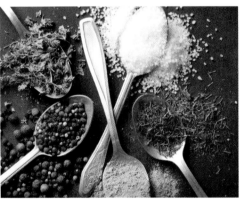
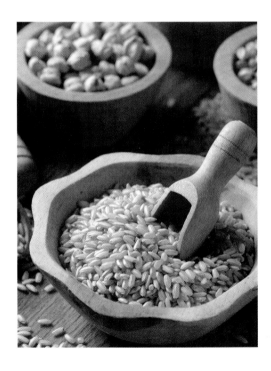
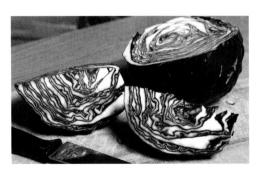

DAY 20

FRESH TOMATO SALSA
Yield: 3 cups

In the summertime when tomato production peaks, it's hard to resist the appeal of fresh salsa. It gets better after it has time to linger in the fridge. This recipe is not too hot or too mild but just right.

> 2 large tomatoes, cored and diced
> ½ red onion, peeled and diced
> 1 jalapeno pepper, seeded and minced
> Juice of 1 lime
> ½ cup chopped fresh cilantro
> ½ teaspoon garlic salt
> ½ teaspoon black pepper
> ⅛ teaspoon dried cumin

1. Place the tomatoes, diced onion pieces, jalapeno pepper, lime juice, cilantro, salt, pepper, and cumin in a mixing bowl.
2. Stir well, cover, and refrigerate at least 2 hours.
3. When ready to serve, bring to room temperature for at least 15 minutes.

Note: For those who like to pack the heat punch with their salsa, use the same receipe above, except use 2 jalapeno peppers (or 3 if you can handle it!).

FOOD FACT: BEANS

Refrigerate fresh beans in a perforated plastic bag for up to three days in the vegetable crisper. For longer storage, blanch and freeze the beans.

BEAN SALAD WITH LEMON DRESSING
Yield: 4 servings

There is no reason this salad can't be made on a regular basis. It's quick and enormously satisfying thanks to a mildly sweet lemony dressing. It is a great side dish with baked fish. You can use dried beans instead of canned, cooked per the recipe found on page 95.

> 1 lemon, zested and juiced
> 2 tablespoons walnut oil
> 2 tablespoons honey
> 1 garlic clove, peeled and minced
> ¼ teaspoon black pepper
> 1 (14-ounce) can garbanzo beans, drained and rinsed
> 1 (14-ounce) can dark red kidney beans, drained and rinsed
> Mixed salad greens

1. In a jar with a tight-fitting lid, combine the lemon zest, lemon juice, oil, honey, garlic, and pepper. Cover and shake to emulsify. Set aside.
2. In a serving bowl, combine the garbanzo beans, kidney beans, and edamame.
3. Toss with the dressing and cover.
4. Let stand for at least 10 minutes before serving at room temperature over mixed salad greens.

FOOD FACT: ONIONS

Selection: Bulb onions should feel hard and have no signs of green shoots emerging from the cut end.

LEMON BROCCOLI SOUP
Yield: 2 servings

Forget about broccoli soup that is prepared with cream and loads of cheese. This healthy alternative relies on merely a cup of diced potatoes to give it body and lemon juice to keep it fresh.

1 tablespoon extra-virgin oil
1 medium sweet onion, peeled and
    chopped
2 garlic cloves, peeled and minced
1 (10-ounce) package broccoli florets
1 cup finely chopped potato
4 cups vegetable stock (see page 96)
Juice of ½ lemon
¼ teaspoon black pepper
⅛ teaspoon cayenne
2 tablespoons plain Greek yogurt
1 tablespoon chopped fresh chives

1. Place the oil in a deep saucepan or Dutch oven over medium-low heat.
2. When hot, add the chopped onion pieces and sauté 5 minutes, stirring occasionally.
3. Add the garlic and cook 1 minute longer.
4. Add the broccoli, potatoes, and stock. Bring to a boil, then reduce the heat to low. Cover and simmer 25 minutes.
5. With an immersion blender, puree the soup until smooth.
6. Stir in the lemon juice, pepper, and cayenne.
7. Ladle into serving bowls and garnish with the yogurt and chives. Serve warm.

FOOD FACT: BROCCOLI

Storage: Broccoli likes the crisper drawer in the refrigerator and if it is in a plastic bag, make sure it is loosely closed.

Lime-Infused Black Bean Salad
Yield: 4 servings

Between the lime juice and cilantro, this salad packs a real zing! It is absolutely gorgeous and benefits from time in the refrigerator. Use shoepeg corn in this recipe if you can.

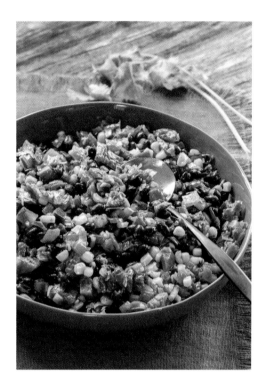

2 tablespoons extra-virgin oil

1 purple onion, peeled and chopped

2 garlic cloves, peeled and minced

2 (15-ounce) cans black beans, drained and rinsed

2 large tomatoes, chopped (seeded if desired)

2 cups whole kernel corn

½ cup chopped fresh cilantro

2½ tablespoons lime juice

1 tablespoon extra-virgin oil

1 teaspoon ground cumin

½ teaspoon sugar

½ teaspoon salt

¼ teaspoon black pepper

¼ teaspoon hot sauce

Mixed salad greens

1. Place the oil in a large skillet over medium heat.

2. When hot, add the chopped onion pieces and cook, stirring frequently for 4 minutes.

3. Add the garlic and cook 1 minute longer, stirring constantly. Remove from the heat and set aside to cool slightly.

4. Meanwhile, in a large bowl, combine the black beans, tomatoes, corn, and cilantro.

5. In a small bowl, whisk together the lime juice, olive oil, cumin, sugar, salt, pepper, and hot sauce.

6. Pour over the tomato mixture and toss to evenly coat.

7. Add the onion mixture and mix well. Cover and refrigerate at least 2 hours.

8. When ready to serve, remove from the refrigerator for 30 minutes. Toss again and serve over mixed salad greens.

Fresh Tomato Basil Soup
Yield: 4 servings

Who doesn't love tomato soup on a chilly day? If you don't puree it with an immersion blender, the taste changes completely. You will like both versions!

2 tablespoons extra-virgin oil
1 large sweet onion, peeled and
    chopped
4 garlic cloves, peeled and minced
2 carrots, peeled and sliced
1 celery stalk, chopped
4 cups low sodium organic vegetable or
    chicken stock (see page 96 or 117)
3½ cups chopped tomatoes
    (seeded if desired)
2 teaspoons red wine vinegar
½ teaspoon salt
½ teaspoon black pepper
16 large, fresh basil leaves, divided

1. Place the oil in a Dutch oven over medium heat.
2. When hot, add the chopped onion pieces and cook, stirring frequently for 3 minutes.
3. Add the garlic and cook 1 minute longer, stirring constantly.
4. Stir in the carrots and celery and reduce the heat to low. Cover and cook 12 minutes.
5. Add the stock, tomatoes, basil, vinegar, salt, and pepper. Increase the heat to medium-high and bring to a boil.
6. Reduce the heat to low and simmer uncovered for 10 minutes.
7. Stir in 12 of the basil leaves during the last 2 minutes of cooking.
8. Remove from the heat and with an immersion blender, puree the soup until smooth (optional). Chop the remaining basil and garnish. Serve warm.

Brown Rice & Berry Pilaf
Yield: 3 servings

This is a terrific side dish for turkey, but you can use it in so many different ways. It can be a wrap filling or you can increase the amount of cabbage and serve it as a salad.

1 tablespoon extra-virgin oil
1 shallot, peeled and chopped
1 celery stalk, chopped
⅔ cup brown rice
2 cups warm chicken stock
    (see page 117)
½ small head of cabbage,
    shredded
3 tablespoons dried cranberries
¼ cup toasted chopped walnuts
3 tablespoons snipped fresh chives
¼ teaspoon cracked black pepper

1. Place the oil in a large frying pan over high heat.
2. Add the chopped shallot pieces and celery and cook, stirring frequently, for 2 minutes.

3. Add the rice and cook another 2 minutes, stirring frequently.
4. Add the stock and bring to a boil. Reduce the heat to medium and cover. Cook for 10 minutes.
5. Place the cabbage on top of the rice, cover, and reduce the heat to low. Cook 15-17 minutes or until the rice is tender and the cabbage is cooked.
6. Add the cranberries and walnuts during the last 2 minutes of cooking.
7. Garnish with the chives and pepper and serve warm.

FOOD FACT: WALNUTS

Storage: Unshelled walnuts can be stored in a cool, dry place up to three months. Don't shell them until you are ready to use. Shelled walnuts can be stored in the refrigerator up to six months or up to one year in the freezer.

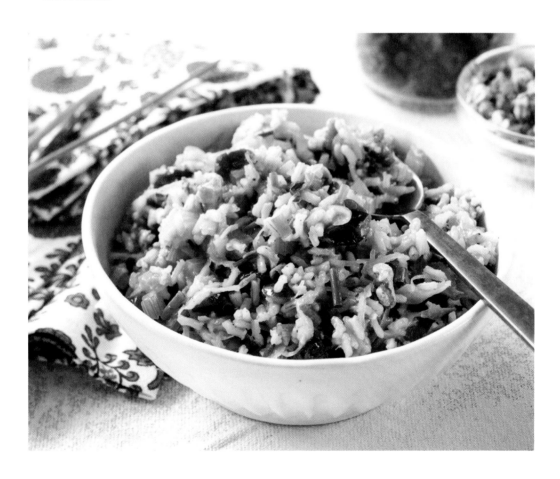

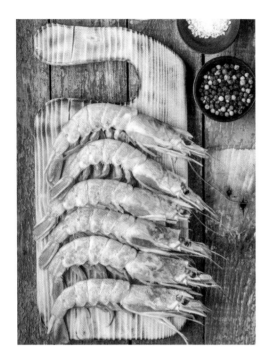
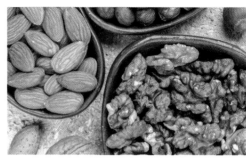
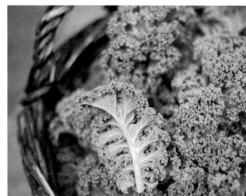
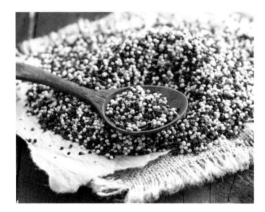
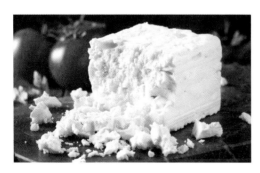
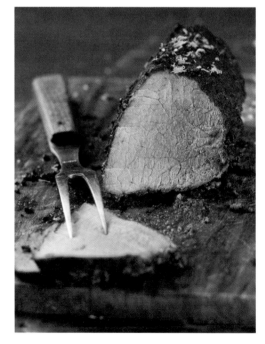

DAY 21

GRILLED PEACH & SHRIMP SALAD
Yield: 2 servings

Purchase the largest shrimp you can find for this impressive main dish salad. It cooks quickly, so have all the other steps ready to serve. No grill? No problem! Just substitute lump crabmeat for the shrimp and use the peaches raw.

1 pound jumbo raw shrimp, peeled
    and deveined
3 tablespoons extra-virgin oil, divided
2 large peaches, peeled, seeded,
    and cut in wedges
Mixed salad greens
¼ teaspoon salt
⅛ teaspoon black pepper
2 tablespoons balsamic vinegar
8 whole roasted walnuts or pecans
Shaved Parmesan or crumbled Feta
    for garnish

1. Preheat the grill to medium-high.
2. Thread the shrimp on skewers and brush with 1 tablespoon of olive oil.
3. Thread the peach wedges on separate skewers.
4. Grill 2 minutes on each side.
   Note: The shrimp might need an extra minute. Grill just until they turn pink.
5. Place the salad greens in a serving bowl and add the salt and pepper.
6. Toss with the remaining oil and vinegar. Add the shrimp and peaches and top with the pecans.
7. Garnish with the cheese and serve immediately.

FOOD FACT: PEACHES

Ripening: I like to buy peaches at various stages of ripeness so they aren't all ready to use at the same time. If your peaches are hard and you need them to soften, place in a paper bag and close loosely. Let stand at room temperature for a few days and check the bag daily for progress.

ROAST BEEF & QUINOA WRAPS
Yield: 2 servings

These wraps utilize leftover roast beef, but you can certainly incorporate any protein you wish. The pear is the secret ingredient!

1 pear, peeled, cored, and finely
   chopped
1 tablespoon lemon juice
1 small shallot, peeled and chopped
2 cups shredded cooked roast beef,
   room temperature
1 cup cooked quinoa, room temperature
1 cup shredded lettuce
2 tablespoons pine nuts
2 (10-inch) gluten-free, whole wheat, or
   organic corn tortillas

1. Place the chopped pear pieces in
   a mixing bowl and toss with the
   lemon juice.
2. Add the chopped shallot pieces, roast
   beef, quinoa, lettuce, and pine nuts.
3. Place the tortillas on a cutting board and
   divide the mixture evenly on top.
4. Roll tightly and secure with toothpicks if
   necessary. Serve immediately.

FOOD FACT: PEARS

Speedy Ripening: If you need pears
to ripen faster than they would naturally, place them in a closed brown
paper bag and leave them in a cool,
dark place like your pantry. This
traps the naturally occurring eth-
ylene gas and helps the pear soften
for quick use.

GOLDEN RAISIN BRAN MUFFINS
Yield: about 12 muffins

Need a reason to rise and shine? This is it!
Making a simple switch from regular dark
to golden raisins gives these muffins a great
flavor with plump, juicy raisins in each bite.

1 cup gluten-free all-purpose flour
¾ cup bran
½ cup whole wheat flour (or 1½ cup
   gluten-free all-purpose flour
   if entirely gluten-free)
2 teaspoons baking powder
1 teaspoon ground cinnamon
½ teaspoon baking soda
½ teaspoon salt
1¼ cups almond, coconut, or nonfat milk
½ cup packed light brown sugar
⅓ cup extra-virgin oil
2 teaspoons apple cider vinegar
1 teaspoon pure vanilla extract
⅔ cup golden raisins

1. Preheat the oven to 400 degrees.
2. Line 12 muffin cups with paper liners
   and set aside.
3. In a mixing bowl, stir together the
   all-purpose flour, bran, wheat flour,
   baking powder, cinnamon, baking soda,
   and salt.
4. In a separate bowl, whisk together the
   milk, sugar, oil, vinegar, and extract.
5. Add to the flour mixture and stir just
   until blended.

6. Fold in the raisins and evenly divide the batter among the muffin cups.
7. Bake for 18-20 minutes or until a cake tester inserted in the center comes out clean.
8. Let cool in the pan on a wire rack for 3 minutes. Remove from the pan and cool completely on the rack.

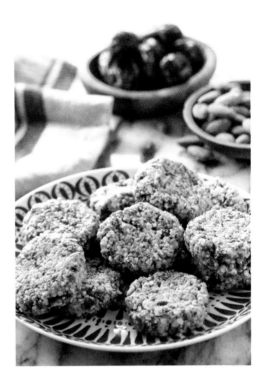

FOOD FACT: ALMONDS

Almonds are one of the foods known to lower blood sugar, prevent memory loss, relieve ADHD and autism, and decrease anxiety.

NO-BAKE ALMOND COOKIES
Yield: about 12 cookies

This is a great and nutritional recipe to satisfy a sweet craving. It doesn't require the heat of an oven, just a food processor. And it makes less than a dozen cookies, so there aren't lots to hang around for a long period of time.

1 cup whole almonds
1 cup pitted dates
½ cup almond butter
½ teaspoon pure almond extract
Pinch of salt

1. Place the whole almonds in the bowl of a food processor and pulse into flour.
2. Add the dates, almond butter, extract, and salt to the processor.
3. Process until the dough is crumbly.
4. Form into balls and gently press down onto a sheet pan covered in waxed paper.
5. Make indentions with a fork and refrigerate at least 8 hours before serving.

GRILLED MUSHROOMS ON ROSEMARY SKEWERS
Yield: 2 servings

Forget soaking wood skewers. Just strip the leaves off rosemary stems, and you've got a sturdy grilling stick that is loaded with aroma and flavor. They cook so quickly that you can add the threaded stems to the already fired-up grill. Feel free to use any type of mushroom you like.

- 1 tablespoon extra-virgin oil
- 1 tablespoon lemon juice
- 1 tablespoon balsamic vinegar
- ¼ teaspoon salt
- ¼ teaspoon black pepper
- ⅛ teaspoon cayenne
- 1 (8-ounce) package whole cremini mushrooms, washed
- 4 stripped rosemary stems

1. In a small bowl, whisk together the oil, juice, vinegar, salt, pepper, and cayenne.
2. Place the mushrooms in a zip-top bag and add the marinade. Seal and allow to stand at room temperature for 1 hour.
3. Preheat the grill to medium-high.
4. Thread the mushrooms onto the rosemary by twisting them onto the stems.
5. Transfer any leftover marinade to a small bowl.
6. Place the skewers on the grate and grill for 3 to 4 minutes, turning halfway through and basting with the leftover marinade.
7. Place on parchment paper and seal up into a packet. Allow to stand 5 minutes before serving warm or at room temperature.

FOOD FACT: PEPPERS

Keep your hands away from your lips and eyes when working with peppers. Make sure and wash your hands thoroughly with soap and water immediately after handling peppers.

KALE POSOLE
Yield: 6 servings

You can certainly add cooked chicken or turkey to this thick stew, but it really isn't needed. The hominy and chickpeas give it all the depth it needs, and the chopped green kale tops it off deliciously. You can substitute Anaheim for the poblano chili, if desired.

- 2 teaspoons extra-virgin oil
- 1 sweet onion, peeled and diced
- 1 poblano or Anaheim chili pepper, seeded and minced
- 3 garlic cloves, peeled and minced

2 (15.5-ounce) cans chickpeas, drained and rinsed

1 (15.5-ounce) can white hominy, drained and rinsed

1 large tomato, diced

3 cups low sodium vegetable stock (see page 96)

2 cups chopped fresh kale

½ teaspoon salt

¼ teaspoon black pepper

1. Place the oil in a Dutch oven over medium-high heat.

2. When hot, add the diced onion pieces, chili pepper, and garlic. Cook, stirring constantly for 1 minute.

3. Add the chickpeas, hominy, and diced tomato. Add just enough stock to cover the mixture. Bring to a boil, reduce the heat to low, and cover. Simmer 20 minutes.

4. Remove from the heat and stir in the kale, salt, and pepper. Allow to stand covered for 2 minutes. Serve warm.

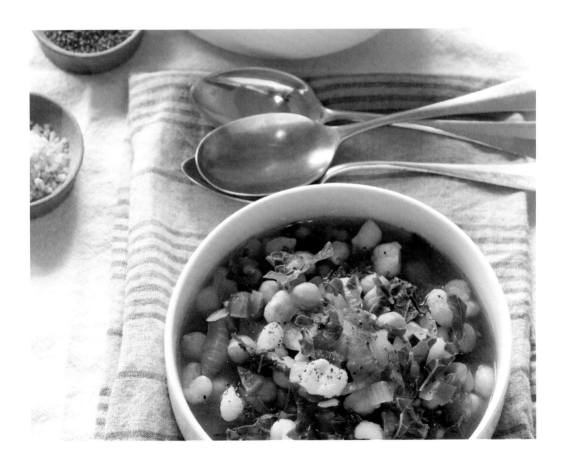

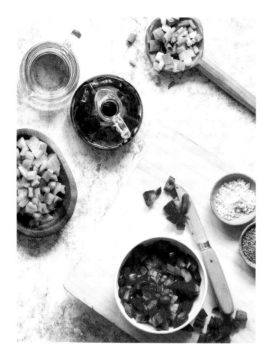

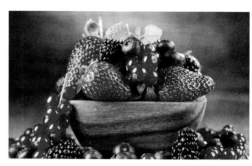

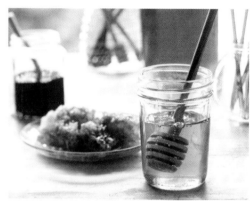

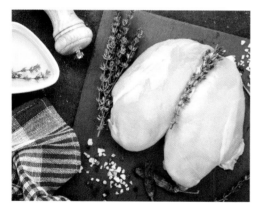

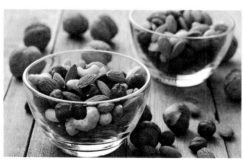

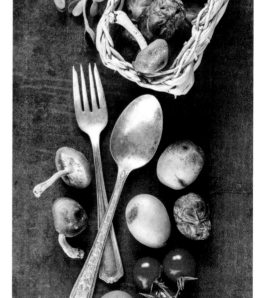

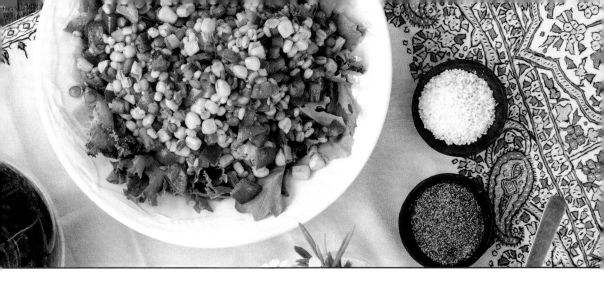

APPENDIX

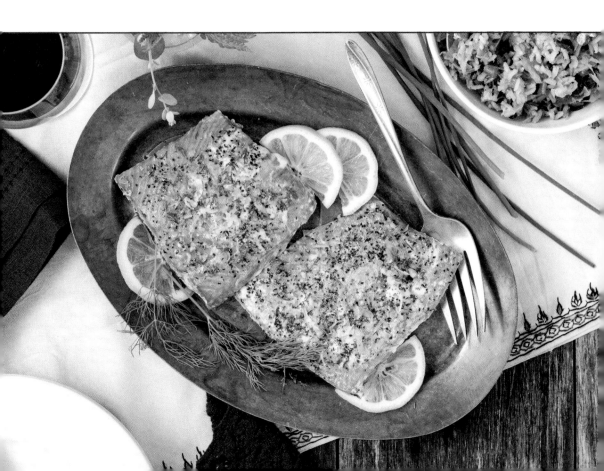

APPENDIX A: SHOPPING LISTS

SHOPPING LIST – STAPLES

FRUITS

- ☐ Apples (Granny Smith) – 3-pound bag
- ☐ Lemons – 2-pound bag
- ☐ Limes – 2-pound bag

VEGETABLES

- ☐ Beets – 1 bunch
- ☐ Celery – 1 bunch
- ☐ Carrots – 2-pound bag (whole)
- ☐ Garlic – 3-ounce package fresh or 4.5-ounce jar
- ☐ Jicama – 1 pound
- ☐ Mint – 1 bunch
- ☐ Onions – 2-pound bag
- ☐ Parsley – 1 bunch
- ☐ Parsnips – 1-pound bag
- ☐ Potatoes – 2-pound bag
- ☐ Radish – 1
- ☐ Shallots – 3-ounce package
- ☐ Sweet Potatoes – 2-pound bag
- ☐ Turnips** – 1 pound
- ☐ Winter Squash** – 2-pounds

OILS AND VINEGARS

- ☐ Extra-Virgin Olive, Avocado, or Coconut Oil – 16-ounce bottle
- ☐ Balsamic Vinegar – 16-ounce bottle
- ☐ Apple Cider Vinegar – 16-ounce bottle

NUTS AND SEEDS

- ☐ Almonds – 1-pound (whole)
- ☐ Cashews – 1-pound (whole)
- ☐ Macadamia Nuts – 10-ounces
- ☐ Peanuts – 1-pound jar (unsalted)
- ☐ Pecans – 1 pound (whole)
- ☐ Pistachio Nuts – 1 pound
- ☐ Pumpkin Seeds – 10-ounces (unsaltcd)
- ☐ Sunflower Seeds – 8-ounces (unsalted)
- ☐ Walnuts – 1 pound (whole)

GRAINS

- ☐ Brown Rice – 10-ounce package
- ☐ Gluten–Free Bread – 12-ounce loaf*
- ☐ Gluten–Free Bagels – 14-ounce package*
- ☐ Gluten–Free Pita Bread – 19-ounce package*
- ☐ Gluten–Free Tortillas – 14-ounce package†
- ☐ Gluten–Free Granola – 12-ounce package
- ☐ Gluten–Free Quinoa – 15-ounce package
- ☐ Gluten–Free Rice Noodles – 8-ounce package
- ☐ Chia Seeds – 1 pound
- ☐ Flaxseeds – 1 pound

DAIRY/EGGS

- [ ] Coconut or Almond Milk
  – 1 gallon every other week
- [ ] Organic Eggs – 1 dozen
- [ ] Parmesan Cheese
  – ¼-pound wedge
- [ ] Feta Cheese – 6-ounce container
- [ ] Organic Butter – 1 pound
- [ ] Plain Greek Yogurt
  – 1 32-ounce container

CANNED AND PACKAGED

- [ ] Green Tea – 40 tea bags
- [ ] Coffee – 30.5-ounce container
- [ ] Sparkling Water – 6 (16-ounce) bottles
- [ ] Tea – 15 tea bag package
- [ ] Stevia – 16-ounce package
- [ ] Red Beans – 1 dried package or 10-ounce can
- [ ] Black Beans – 2 dried packages or 2 10-ounce cans
- [ ] Northern or White Beans
  – 1 dried package or 10-ounce can
- [ ] Lima Beans – 1 dried package or 10-ounce can
- [ ] Smart Balance Light Mayonnaise
  – 16-ounce jar
- [ ] Plant Protein Powder
  – 1-pound container
- [ ] Cashew Nut Butter
  – 8-ounce jar†
- [ ] Almond Nut Butter
  – 8-ounce jar†
- [ ] Gluten–Free Peanut Butter
  – 8-ounce jar

- [ ] Steel-Cut Oatmeal
  – 16-ounce package*
- [ ] Buck Wheat Flour – 1 package
- [ ] Gluten-Free All Purpose Flour
  – 1 Package
- [ ] Black Bean Soup – 2 19-ounce cans
  or homemade (frozen in ½–1 cup
  portions & thawed)
- [ ] Split Pea, Lentil, or Minestrone Soup
  – 4 19-ounce cans
  or homemade (frozen in
  ½–1 cup portions & thawed)
- [ ] Vegetable Soup – 5 19 oz cans or
  homemade (frozen in
  ½–1 cup portions & thawed)

FROZEN

- [ ] Turkey Bacon – 16-ounce package,
  divided and frozen
- [ ] Veggie Burgers
  – 8-ounce package
- [ ] Turkey Burgers
  – 8-ounce package
- [ ] Edamame – 2 16-ounce packages
- [ ] Pearl Onions
  – 8-ounce package
- [ ] Gluten–Free Pancakes
  – 8–10-ounce package
- [ ] Frozen Fruit – 14-ounce package
  of your choice

† *stored in refrigerator*
* *stored in freezer*
** *when seasonally available*

SHOPPING LIST – WEEK 1

(DAYS 1–7)

FRUITS

- ☐ Apricot – 1
- ☐ Bananas – 4
- ☐ Blueberries – 6-ounce package
- ☐ Cantaloupe or Honeydew – 1
- ☐ Grapefruit – 1 small
- ☐ Kiwi – 1
- ☐ Pear – 1
- ☐ Raspberries – 6-ounce package
- ☐ Seedless Grapes or Cherries – 1 small bag
- ☐ Strawberries – 16-ounce package
- ☐ Watermelon – 1 small

VEGETABLES

- ☐ Asparagus – 3 bunches
- ☐ Avocadoes – 3
- ☐ Bean Sprouts – 4-ounce package
- ☐ Broccoli – 7 day supply
- ☐ Cabbage – 1 head
- ☐ Cauliflower – 2 heads
- ☐ Corn – 1 ear
- ☐ Cucumbers – 7 day supply
- ☐ Eggplant – 2
- ☐ English Peas – 1 serving size
- ☐ Green Beans – 7 day supply
- ☐ Kale – 7 day supply
- ☐ Mushrooms – 7 day supply
- ☐ Peppers (variety of colors) – 7 day supply

- ☐ Pimentos – 1 small jar
- ☐ Salad Greens (chicory, spinach, kale, Belgian endive, bean sprouts, iceberg, romaine) – 7 day supply for twice daily salads
- ☐ Spaghetti Squash – 1 small
- ☐ Summer (Yellow, Zucchini) or Winter (Acorn, Butternut) Squash – 7 day supply
- ☐ Tomatoes – 7 day supply
- ☐ Zucchini – 4 medium size

MEAT

- ☐ Boneless, Skinless Chicken Breast – 2*
- ☐ Crab Meat*
- ☐ Extra Lean Beef (96/4, petite fillet)*
- ☐ Flounder*
- ☐ Mackerel*
- ☐ Salmon Fillet*
- ☐ Shrimp (large)*
- ☐ Turkey Breast Tenderloin – 4*
- ☐ Whitefish Fillet*

amount varies by gender (see meal plan)

SHOPPING LIST — WEEK 2

(DAYS 8–14)

FRUIT

- ☐ Bananas – 4
- ☐ Blackberries – 6-ounce package
- ☐ Blueberries – 6-ounce package
- ☐ Fig – 1
- ☐ Grapefruit – 1
- ☐ Mango – 1
- ☐ Nectarine or Peach – 1
- ☐ Pineapple – 1 small
- ☐ Plum or Tangerine – 1
- ☐ Strawberries – 16-ounce package

VEGETABLES

- ☐ Avocados – 2
- ☐ Broccoli – 7 day supply
- ☐ Brussels Sprouts – 1 serving size
- ☐ Cucumbers – 7 day supply
- ☐ Eggplant – 2
- ☐ English Peas – 1 serving size
- ☐ Fennel – 1 bulb
- ☐ Green Beans – 7 day supply
- ☐ Mushrooms – 7 day supply
- ☐ Okra – 1 serving size
- ☐ Peppers (variety of colors) – 7 day supply
- ☐ Salad Greens (chicory, spinach, kale, Belgian endive, bean sprouts, iceberg, romaine) – 7 day supply for twice daily salads

- ☐ Spinach – 7 day supply
- ☐ Sugar Snap Peas – 1 serving size
- ☐ Swiss Chard – 1 serving size bunch
- ☐ Tomatoes – 7 day supply

CANNED & PACKAGED

- ☐ Hummus – 6-ounce container

MEAT

- ☐ Boneless, Skinless Chicken Breast – 5*
- ☐ Extra Lean Beef (96/4, petite fillet) – 2*
- ☐ Catfish Fillet*
- ☐ Crawfish*
- ☐ Shrimp (large)*
- ☐ Salmon Fillet*
- ☐ Scallops*
- ☐ Tilapia Fillet*
- ☐ Turkey Breast Tenderloin*

amount varies by gender (see meal plan)

SHOPPING LIST – WEEK 3

(DAYS 15–21)

FRUIT
- [ ] Banana – 1
- [ ] Blackberries – 6-ounce container
- [ ] Blueberries – 6-ounce container
- [ ] Clementine or Tangerine – 1
- [ ] Grapefruit – 1
- [ ] Grapes – 1 small bunch
- [ ] Kiwi – 1
- [ ] Papaya or Mango – 1
- [ ] Pear or Pomegranate – 1
- [ ] Tangarine or Orange – 1
- [ ] Strawberries – 16-ounce container

VEGETABLES
- [ ] Asparagus – 3 bunches
- [ ] Broccoli – 7 day supply
- [ ] Cauliflower – 2 heads
- [ ] Corn – 1 ear
- [ ] Cucumbers – 7 day supply
- [ ] Eggplant – 2
- [ ] Green Beans – 7 day supply
- [ ] Leeks – 1 bunch
- [ ] Mushrooms – 7 day supply
- [ ] Okra – 1 serving size
- [ ] Pattypan or Yellow Squash – 2 medium
- [ ] Peppers (variety of colors) – 7 day supply
- [ ] Portabella Mushrooms – 2 large
- [ ] Salad Greens (chicory, spinach, kale, Belgian endive, bean sprouts, iceberg, romaine) – 7 day supply for twice daily salads
- [ ] Snow Peas – 1 serving size
- [ ] Turnip Greens or Bok Choy – 1 bunch
- [ ] Tomatillos – 3 (for salsa)
- [ ] Zucchini – 2 medium

MEAT
- [ ] Boneless, Skinless Chicken Breast*
- [ ] Catfish Fillet*
- [ ] Salmon Fillet*
- [ ] Shrimp (large)*
- [ ] Extra Lean Beef (96/4, petite fillet) *
- [ ] Ground Turkey *
- [ ] Trout Fillet*
- [ ] Tuna *
- [ ] Turkey Breast Tenderloin – 3*
- [ ] White Fish *

amount varies by gender (see meal plan)

APPENDIX B

SUPPLEMENTS

Depending on your health and your sickness, I may suggest one or more supplements to help speed you along the trail toward health. All supplements are recommendations. To review the supplements, go to drcolbert.com. You can order at any time.

Divine Health Nutritional Products
shop.drcolbert.com
407-732-6952

1. Green Supremefood: A whole food nutritional powder with fermented grasses and vegetables
2. Red Supremefood: A whole food nutritional powder with anti-aging fruits
3. Fermented Plant Protein
4. Enhanced Multivitamin

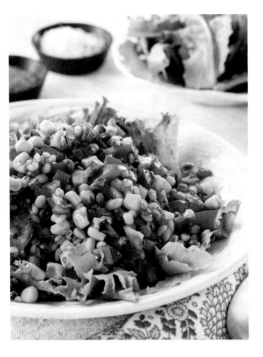

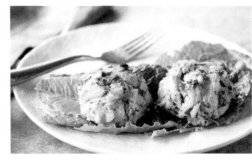

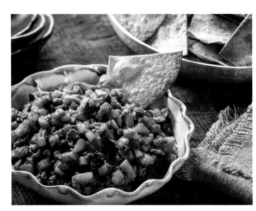

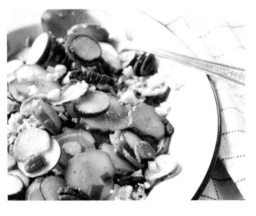

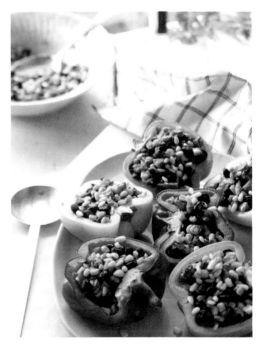

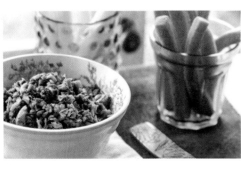

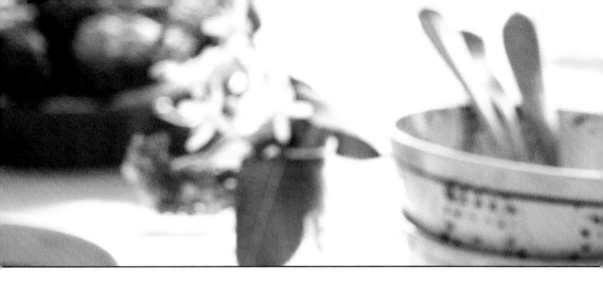

INDEX

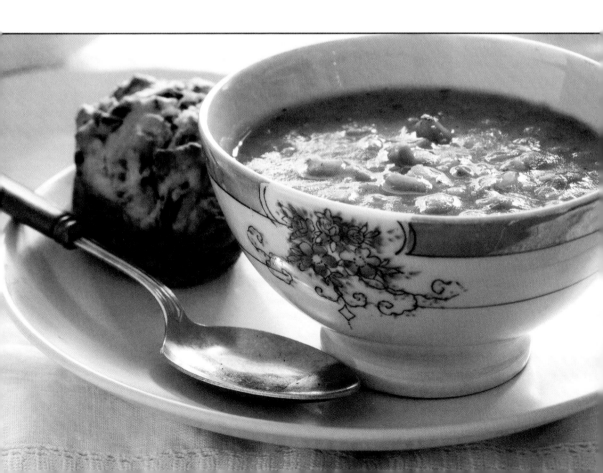

RECIPE INDEX

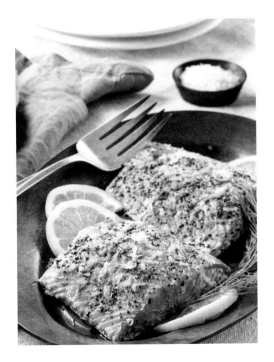

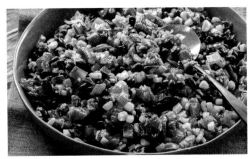

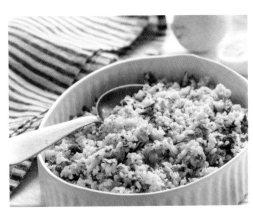

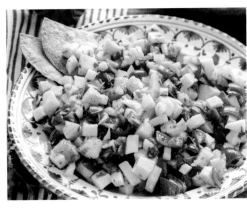

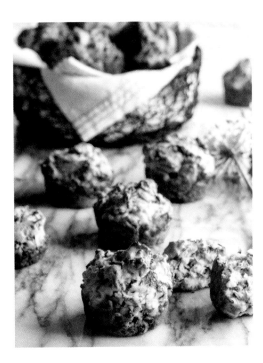

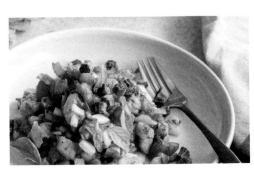

ABOUT THE AUTHOR

DON COLBERT, MD graduated from Oral Roberts University Medical School in 1984. He then moved to Central Florida, where he did his internship and residency at Florida Hospital. For over twenty-five years, Dr. Colbert has practiced medicine in Central Florida. He has been board certified in family practice for over twenty-five years and specializes in anti-aging medicine. Dr. Colbert is also a *New York Times* best-selling author who has written more than forty books.

Dr. Colbert has ministered health and healing to thousands. He is a frequent guest with John Hagee, Joyce Meyer, Kenneth Copeland, James Robison, Jim Bakker, and other leaders in the body of Christ. Dr. Colbert has also been featured on *The Dr. Oz Show*, Fox News, ABC World News, BBC and in *Readers Digest*, *News Week*, *Prevention* magazine, and many others.

Dr. Colbert offers seminars and talks on a variety of topics including "How to Improve Your Health," "The Effects of Stress and How to Overcome It," "Deadly Emotions," and "The Seven Pillars of Health." Through his research and walk with God, Dr. Colbert has been given a unique insight that has helped thousands improve their lives.

To contact Dr. Colbert's office, you can do so via:

Internet: drcolbert.com
Phone: 407-331-7007
Fax: 407-331-5777
Email: info@drcolbert.com
Facebook: facebook.com/DonColbertMD
Twitter: @DonColbert

CHOOSING A BETTER LIFE
ONE MEAL AT A TIME

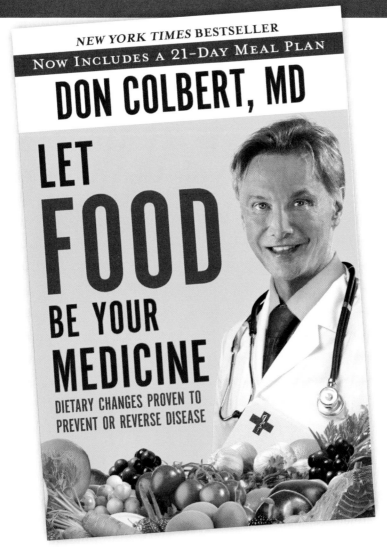

NEW YORK TIMES BESTSELLER

NOW INCLUDES A 21-DAY MEAL PLAN

DON COLBERT, MD

LET
FOOD
BE YOUR
MEDICINE

DIETARY CHANGES PROVEN TO
PREVENT OR REVERSE DISEASE

DISCOVER AN APPROACH TO NUTRITION
THAT WILL CHANGE YOUR HEALTH AND LIFE FOREVER

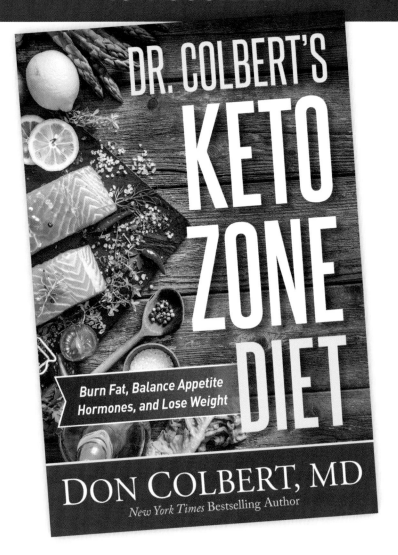

IF YOU ENJOYED THIS BOOK, WILL YOU CONSIDER SHARING THE MESSAGE WITH OTHERS?

Mention the book in a blog post or through Facebook, Twitter, Pinterest, or upload a picture through Instagram.

Recommend this book to those in your small group, book club, workplace, and classes.

Head over to facebook.com/DonColbertMD, "LIKE" the page, and post a comment as to what you enjoyed the most.

Tweet "I recommend reading #LetFoodBeYourMedicineCookbook by @DonColbert // @worthypub"

Pick up a copy for someone you know who would be challenged and encouraged by this message.

Write a book review online.

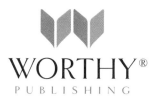

Visit us at worthypublishing.com

twitter.com/worthypub

instagram.com/worthypub

facebook.com/worthypublishing

youtube.com/worthypublishing